T0210144

High Volume
Spay AND Neuter

A Safe and Time Efficient Approach

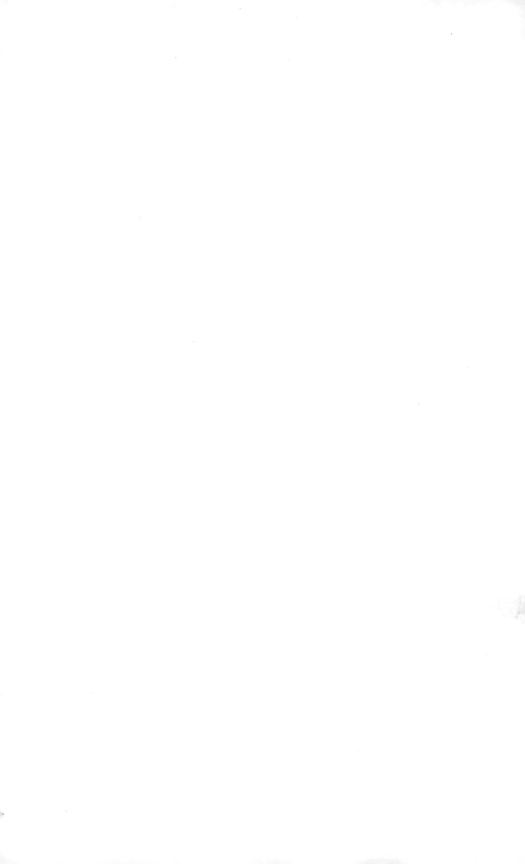

High Volume Spay AND Neuter

A Safe and Time Efficient Approach

VICTORIA VALDEZ, DVM

Medical Director 2012–2018
Spay-4-LA
Mobile Spay/Neuter Clinic
Los Angeles, CA, USA

ELSEVIER

Elsevier
1600 John F. Kennedy Blvd.
Ste 1800
Philadelphia, PA 19103-2899

Notice

Library of Congress Control Number: 2021933380

Senior Content Strategist: Jennifer Catando (Flynn-Briggs)
Content Development Manager: Meghan Andress
Content Development Specialist: Kevin Travers
Publishing Services Manager: Deepthi Unni
Senior Project Manager: Manchu Mohan
Design Direction: Renee Duenow

Printed in the United States of America.

Last digit is the print number: 9 8 7 6 5 4 3 2 1

Working together
to grow libraries in
developing countries

ELSEVIER   Book Aid
International

www.elsevier.com • www.bookaid.org

This volume is dedicated to my father,
Rudy Valdez,
who began instilling in me a love of books
even before I could talk.

ACKNOWLEDGMENTS

Over the last 10 years, I have had the privilege to work with some wonderful organizations and individuals in the Southern California high-volume spay/neuter community.

The first spay/neuter relief job I had was with Angel Dogs. Thank you to Lisa Tipton for taking a chance with me and referring me to the nonprofit, Spay-4-LA, where I worked full time for the next 8 years and was the medical director for 6 years.

Thanks to everyone at Spay-4-LA for seeing me through my growing pains. A special thank you to all the lay staff and especially to my manager, Sandy Sagastume.

I'd like to express my appreciation to my friend, Karn Myers, who owns FixNation, a state-of-the-art, nonprofit facility for the spay/neuter of feral cats, and all the doctors who work there to combat cat overpopulation. While at FixNation, I learned to do an autoligation feline spay. Thank you to Dr. Yikcia (Milanes) Pope for sharing her knowledge of this technique with me. A special thank you to Dr. Kate Creighton, who taught me how to assess the gestational ages of feline fetuses, and Dr. Derek Turner, who taught me how to tie a Miller's knot. On behalf of all the cats you have helped, I applaud everyone on staff at FixNation.

Working at the shelter run by Riverside County, Department of Animal Services, has given me a broader understanding of the unique challenges that confront a government-owned facility and the outstanding job that this organization does. A shout-out to the staff for their dedication and the great job they do. Special thanks to head veterinarian, Sara Strongin, and my immediate supervisor, Katherine Buff.

In between and to supplement the above positions, I have often done relief work at other facilities such as Spay/Neuter Project, LA, Humane Society of San Bernardino, Mary S. Roberts, Pet Adoption Center, and others. Thank you to those facilities. I have learned valuable information everywhere I have worked.

Through these facilities, I have worked with numerous pet rescue organizations whose efforts on the part of homeless animals are no less than herculean. It takes all of us working together to make any appreciable headway in the fight to combat pet overpopulation and the inherent animal suffering it fosters.

Thank you to all who fight for those who cannot fight for themselves.

Victoria Valdez, DVM

CONTENTS

High Volume
Spay AND Neuter
A Safe and Time Efficient Approach

Fundamentals

CHAPTER 1

Introduction

Victoria Valdez, DVM

When I first went to work full-time in a high-volume spay/neuter practice in 2010, I went to work for a brand-new mobile practice. It was fortunate that this was a new practice and that it took time to build clientele, because frankly, I had no idea how to do 30 sterilization surgeries in a day.

No one on the staff or in management knew how to do that either. We all just assumed we had to work really fast and that we would get faster with experience. Fortunately, we all worked well together and were able to, by trial and error, develop a system that worked well for us, and in time we were able to do 30 and more surgeries in a day, safely and efficiently.

I searched the internet for books on high-volume spay/neuter and found none at that time. I was the only doctor on the mobile unit, so I had no colleagues to consult as problems presented. When I was starting out, I wondered how I could increase my speed without compromising patient safety. In those early days, when complications occurred, I wondered how I could have avoided them and if other veterinarians encountered the same problems. Thankfully, I was also working part-time at an all-cat high-volume spay/neuter practice that specialized in feral cats, and at that practice there were some wonderful veterinarians that shared their knowledge with me. With their help, and the knowledge I gained in the ensuing years, I developed a system that works for me. Since there seems to be a dearth of volumes devoted to this topic, I felt the need to write about my experiences and what I have learned. Texts on standard, full-service spay and neuter surgeries, written by board-certified surgeons, are invaluable as a source of information on good surgical technique. These texts do not, however, address the unique needs of a high-volume spay/neuter practice. With more and more animal welfare organizations, animal control agencies, and animal rescue groups turning to high-volume spay/neuter as a means to control animal over-population and improve the lives of our companion animals, I felt that a text devoted solely to this topic was much needed.

I have had over ten years of experience doing high volume spay/neuter. I was the medical director and surgeon for a mobile, non-profit spay/neuter clinic for eight years. I also worked part-time, for many years, for an all feline (primarily feral) non-profit spay/neuter clinic, and a large Southern California county animal shelter. I have also worked relief for a number of rescue organizations. My experience has been varied and extensive. I have done over 60,000 spays and neuters.

My goal is to pass on what I have learned regarding this challenging area of practice. The ideas presented here do not, by any means, encompass the only way to organize or execute a high-volume spay/neuter practice. They are what works for me. They have evolved over many years, and I am sure they will continue to change and improve as new ideas, equipment, and techniques become available. If you are happy with what you are doing, you should continue doing it; if not, I hope that you can use these techniques as a starting point or incorporate some or all of them into what you are currently doing.

I have written this book with the hope that it will be used as a reference. For that reason, there is some repetition from chapter to chapter. I did this so that the reader can go to a chapter dealing with a specific topic and get all the information needed on that topic, without the need to flip back and forth to other chapters. I hope you find this helpful.

In Section 2, Surgical Protocols, each protocol includes a section on troubleshooting. This is where problems that can arise during surgery are described and solutions to them are offered. Although a certain problem may be discussed under the protocol for one specific type of surgery, it may well apply to many of the surgery types. For a list of all the troubleshooting topics that are addressed, refer to "Troubleshooting" in the index.

This text is written and directed toward veterinarians interested in high-volume spay/neuter. My hope is that it will also be of value to veterinary support staff in this field. Those groups, such as animal welfare organizations and animal rescue groups, looking to establish a new spay/neuter program or streamline the one they have may also find it helpful. Depending on your level of expertise, some of the things I address here may already be known to you or some may be brand new. To those of you with more experience, please bear with me. This volume is meant to be used by everyone from the new graduate to the seasoned practitioner looking to increase the volume of surgeries he or she performs in a day.

I am always looking for ways to improve what I do, so if you have ideas or techniques you find helpful for high-volume spay/neuter, I would love to hear from you.

CHAPTER 2

Principles of High-Volume Spay/Neuter

Victoria Valdez, DVM

The first question veterinarians new to high-volume spay/neuter always ask is, "How can I get faster?" Unfortunately, when we use words like "faster" and "speed" in the context of high-volume spay/neuter, the image we conjure is one of rushing through a surgery. There is a perception among the public, as well as some full-service veterinarians, that high-volume spay/neuter veterinarians rush through their surgeries, implying that they are sloppy. Nothing could be further from the truth. If a surgeon rushes through procedures, there are bound to be complications. Nothing consumes time like complications, whether it means having to redo something during surgery or having to address a complication via a recheck. Therefore, a high-volume spay/neuter surgeon cannot possibly be "sloppy" and "fast"; the two terms are contradictory.

How then is the demand of high-volume spay/neuter practice met? The name itself indicates that an inordinate number of surgeries are performed in a day. A typical high-volume practice completes an average of 30-plus surgeries a day. This is achieved by a combination of judicious scheduling, clockwork-like teamwork, and overall efficiency.

The primary goal in high-volume spay/neuter practice is to be efficient, that is, to SAFELY perform a sterilization surgery in as little time as possible while doing a QUALITY job. This chapter deals with the principles used in high-volume spay/neuter that directly relate to achieving efficiency. Subsequent chapters will detail how to institute these principles.

PRINCIPLES OF HIGH-VOLUME SPAY/NEUTER

The Purpose of High-Volume Spay/Neuter is Trifold

The purpose of high-volume spay/neuter is trifold: to address the problem of pet overpopulation, to serve an underserved population, and to do so in a fiscally responsible manner.

The many benefits of sterilization of dogs and cats are well documented. Sterilization prior to adoption decreases the number of unwanted pets in shelters and rescue agencies. Controlling the numbers in free-roaming cat populations has many benefits to those cats and to the community.

High-volume spay/neuter makes sterilization available to low-income pet owners. For these owners, the cost of traditional surgery performed at a full-service hospital is often prohibitive.

The only way to serve the high numbers in this demographic in a fiscally sound manner is with a highly efficient program. Since the numbers involved in these scenarios are so high, it is generally more fiscally sound to establish a high-volume spay/neuter program in conjunction with organizations devoted to addressing the problem of homeless pets than it is to avail the services of full-service veterinary practices.

A High-Volume Problem Requires A High-Volume Solution

The numbers of unwanted pets born each year is staggering. If there is any hope of curbing this overpopulation problem, pets need to be sterilized in matching numbers.

The Unique Client Base Associated With High-Volume Spay/Neuter Practice must be Factored into Protocols

High-volume spay/neuter practices serve low-income populations. These clients do not have the financial means to pay emergency fees if complications arise. By necessity, all adults in these households may work, meaning patients are often left unsupervised and/or outdoors postoperatively, putting them at higher risk for complications. Additional measures, such as using stronger suture for these surgeries, should be considered. Elizabethan collars and thorough aftercare instructions are imperative. The use of prophylactic antibiotics is controversial, and a discussion of their use is beyond the scope of this text. However, if you are seeing a lot of rechecks involving infected incisions due to exposure to dirt, you may want to review the pros and cons of their use and consider adding them to your protocol.

Certain Risks are Built into High-Volume Spay/Neuter

Because of time and financial constraints, high-volume spay/neuter patients do not routinely have preop bloodwork done. They do not have intravenous (IV) catheters placed, and they do not receive IV fluids. In young healthy animals this is seldom a problem. A problem arises with young animals with occult disease, or older patients with undiagnosed underlying disease. Since owners in this population often cannot afford a preliminary workup, it becomes a question of risk vs. benefit.

Certain Benefits are Built Into High-Volume Spay/Neuter

The surgeon doing high-volume spay/neuter typically has much more experience doing spays and neuters than the typical general practice veterinarian. He or she is therefore able to do the surgery in less time via a much smaller incision. The smaller incision makes for less pain postoperatively. The shorter surgery time means the patient is under anesthesia for a much shorter time, thereby decreasing anesthetic risk, and making the need for IV catheters and fluids and a preliminary workup less imperative, in most cases. The high-volume spay/neuter surgeon also often has more experience handling any spay/neuter-associated complications that might arise.

The Caseload must be Balanced

The caseload for each day must be realistic. Although the goal is high volume, it is not just about numbers. It is not realistic to expect one surgeon to do 30 large canine spays in a day. On the other hand, 60 feline spays in a day is totally doable. The goal is to schedule a good mix of the different types of sterilization surgeries over the course of a day.

Workstations should be Set up for Maximum Efficiency

Workstations should be in locations and set up such that minimal steps are needed to complete all necessary tasks. All supplies should be within easy reach of the person needing them. There should be a consistent place for all necessary supplies and a clear, concise system for keeping them well stocked.

Doctor and Staff must Work in Concert with Each Other as a Team

No one team member is more important than another. Everyone must help each other. If one team member is overloaded, the others, including the doctor, must help, or the system will break down and efficiency will be lost. Doctors should learn to be as self-sufficient as possible. If the support staff has to stop to help the doctor open a pack of suture, for example, that will delay getting the next patient on the table.

The Surgery Table Should Never be Empty

Patients should flow on and off the table. As one patient comes off the surgery table, another should be put on. Time without a patient on the table is called lag time. Lag time, if extended, can greatly diminish productivity. No matter how fast or efficient a surgeon is, he or she cannot complete a surgery if there is no patient on the table.

Little Things can Add up to Large Amounts of Time Saved

What may seem like trivial details that save only seconds of time can in fact add up to significant time saved. Remember when doing 30 surgeries a day, if 2 minutes a surgery is saved, that adds up to an hour. That hour can be an hour saved in wages, six to eight more surgeries performed, or a shorter working day for you.

The Surgeon's Time Should be Reserved for Surgery

The surgeon has a finite number of hours in his or her working day. If a surgeon averages a surgery every 10 minutes, for example, for every 10 minutes he or she spends doing nonsurgery tasks, that is one fewer surgery that will be done that day. No one else can do the actual surgery. So, for maximum production, as much as is possible, the surgeon should do what only the surgeon can do, i.e., surgery.

Safety Always takes Precedence Over Speed

If the surgeon needs to enlarge an incision, it should be done. If more ligatures are needed, they should be placed. If the patient needs fluids, an IV catheter should be instilled, and fluids given. Trying to save time when these more time-consuming steps are indicated will only end up costing precious time and could compromise the patient. Being safe will always save time in the long run by eliminating those time-consuming preventable complications.

Protocol Changes must Meet Safety Standards

Sometimes this means changes made for time efficiency need to be counterbalanced with steps to improve safety. For example, if a suture pattern involving just one knot is used to save time, that should be counterbalanced by applying a couple extra throws to the knot and applying a drop of glue to it (if it is in the skin) to enhance safety.

Efficiency, not Speed, is what Makes High-Volume Spay/Neuter Possible

It is impossible to do 30 or more surgeries in a day just by going faster. Modifications from standard surgical techniques have to be implemented to make them more efficient. Components such as scheduling, set-up, teamwork, and flow are just as vital as the surgical technique to maintaining productivity. There is no one silver bullet to accomplish this. Instead numerous small details are modified so that as a whole they streamline the working day.

Every Effort should be Made to Make Rechecks Unnecessary

Thirty surgeries in a day is doable in a well-organized high-volume spay/neuter practice, but there is not a lot of time left over for seeing rechecks. One or two rechecks can throw the schedule off balance, and more than one or two can wreak havoc. Adherence to the principles listed here will help to minimize the number of rechecks that are presented and the time they take away from surgery time.

High-Volume Spay/Neuter Surgeons Must be Prepared for Unforeseen Complications

Complications occur despite a surgeon's best efforts. They occur for all surgeons. If the surgeon is prepared when, not if, complications arise, it is easier to stay calm and do what needs to be done.

Nothing Trumps Experience

If you are new to high-volume practice, unless you have had a LOT of experience doing full-service spay/neuter, do not expect to start out doing 30 surgeries a day. Do not expect to do keyhole incisions immediately, and it is unlikely you will do 10-minute spays. Those things come with experience, and there is no substitute for experience. If you are unable or feel uncomfortable gaining on-the-job experience, consider volunteering for a rescue organization. Since they will not be paying you, they will be ahead of the game for ANY surgeries you perform. If you are an employer looking to hire a veterinarian who is NOT experienced in high volume, recognize the limitations and do not overbook, or your doctor will become overwhelmed. Your patience will be rewarded as your surgeon becomes more efficient with experience. In my opinion, the best scenario for a novice spay/neuter veterinarian is when the high-volume practice is brand new. In this case, the number of patients per day and the surgeons, experience can grow in tandem as both are becoming established.

CHAPTER 3

Scheduling

Victoria Valdez, DVM

Many times, scheduling protocols are already set at a preexisting high-volume spay/neuter practice. However, the principles discussed in this chapter may be of value when establishing a new practice or attempting to improve use of time in an existing practice. Since various sterilization surgeries require different amounts of time to complete, the ability to complete 30 surgeries a day is very dependent on how many of each type surgery are scheduled. Doing 30 surgeries of one type is not the same as doing 30 surgeries of another type. It is often impossible to do 30 large canine surgeries in a day. However, it would not be unheard of to do 90 or more feline neuters in a day. All the surgeries in a day are seldom all the same type. In fact, a balanced mix of surgery types is the ultimate goal.

FACTORS TO CONSIDER WHEN SCHEDULING SURGERIES

Predictable Factors

The size and species of patients scheduled for a given day greatly influence the time required to complete that schedule. The fastest surgery is a cat neuter, followed by a cat spay, a small dog spay, and then a large dog spay. We can predict how long each of these routine surgeries takes. We can use that knowledge to attempt to schedule a manageable surgery docket.

Unpredictable Factors

Unfortunately, noting the types of patients scheduled still falls short of measuring all the factors that influence a surgeon's ability to complete a given number of cases in a day. Other, less predictable factors that influence how long it takes to do a given surgery include complications (see Chapters 18 and 19), pregnancy, obesity, cryptorchidism, adhesions due to previous surgery or disease, and/or a fractious temperament. Any of these factors, if present, can and will prolong surgery times. These factors are often not revealed at the time an appointment is made and so cannot reliably be factored in when scheduling. They should, however, be considered when assessing productivity; i.e., if the number of surgeries is fewer than expected for a given day, it may be because some of these problems were encountered. This makes judicious attention to scheduling a manageable case load, based on factors we *do* have control over, even more important.

FACTORS THAT LIMIT THE NUMBER OF SURGERIES THAT CAN BE DONE IN A DAY

Average Surgery Time for Each Sterilization Type

For the purposes of this discussion, average surgery time will be defined as the time (in minutes) it takes the surgeon to do a medium sterilization surgery, i.e., a small canine spay (under 40 lb, 18 kg) and/or a standard-technique feline spay. (This time is measured from the time the patient gets on the table until the time the next patient gets on the table.) The time it takes to do either of these surgeries is similar. They are among the most common surgeries performed in high-volume spay/neuter practice, and the time they require is midrange along the spectrum of surgery types seen. Time several (8–10) small canine spays and average them to determine your AVERAGE SURGERY TIME.

Length of Surgery Time Available Per Day

Multiply the number of surgeon's hours per day by 60 to get the number of minutes in a surgeon's day. An 8-hour day equals 480 minutes. Subtract the average number of minutes before the first patient is on the table (first patient set-up time). The first patient set-up time is usually around 15 minutes. (Yours may vary.) Subtract this number again to allow for getting the first patient on the table after lunch. (Surgeons should set up surgery and then scrub while the first patient is being set up [induced, intubated, and prepped] so that no time is wasted while waiting for that first patient.) If the 30 minutes set-up time is subtracted from 480 minutes, the result is 450 minutes of SURGERY TIME AVAILABLE per 8-hour day. If the surgeon is doing the exams, time used for exams has to be subtracted from SURGERY TIME AVAILABLE, and this will greatly reduce the number of surgeries that can be done in a day.

Examination Time

Receptionists should be trained to ask admission questions, or a questionnaire regarding the patient's current health should be filled out at the time of admission. The person admitting the patient should do a cursory check for a nasal or ocular discharge, trouble breathing, dehydration, or weakness. If any of these things are present, the surgery should be postponed and the patient should be referred for a medical workup.

It is more efficient if exams are not done in the presence of the owners because their questions often slow down the exam time. Staff doing intake should be well trained to answer common questions owners have. It is helpful to have a manual(s) listing common questions and answers on hand that the staff can refer to.

In a typical high-volume spay/neuter practice, the morning is spent on intake, doing exams, and administering premed drugs to the day's patients. In most cases, due to fiscal constraints, presurgical blood work is not available for these patients. The physical exam is the only way to assess their current health and therefore is of utmost importance. On pets that can be handled, a minimum database should include the following:

- Weight and temperature.
- Auscultation of the heart and lungs.
- Examination of the teeth for tartar, infection, and retained deciduous teeth.
- Gender verification and assessment of vulva to check for estrus in canine females.
- Abdominal palpation to check for pregnancy in females.
- Scrotal palpation to check for retained testicles in males.
- Examination of eyes and nose for signs of upper respiratory disease.
- Palpation of the trachea to check for "Kennel Cough" in canines.

Who Does the Examinations

Depending on the laws in the state in which the practice is located, all or some of the exam may be done by a licensed technician. Variations of this include the following:

- The doctor does the entire examination.
- The support staff does only the weight and temp, the doctor does the examination.
- The licensed technician does the examination, the doctor ausculas the heart.
- The licensed technician does the examination and brings any abnormalities to the doctor's attention.
- Only you can determine what works best for your practice.

If the surgeon is doing the examinations, the time it takes to complete these must be subtracted from his or her total surgery time available for the day. It is most productive if the surgeon's time is used for what only the surgeon can do, i.e., surgery. Where state law allows technicians to do examinations, it is most efficient if they are done before the surgeon begins his or her day. (This often necessitates that licensed techs work a 10-hour day so that they can do exams before the surgeon arrives and discharge patients at the end of the day, after the surgeon leaves.)

To determine the time needed for the surgeon to do examinations, time how long is spent on them (including time to premed) each day for several days. Divide that number, in minutes, by the number of patients seen that day to determine how much time per patient is needed for examinations.

The Number of Large Animals Scheduled Per Day

Large or obese female canines are wearing on the surgeon because of the increased difficulty of doing large dog spays. The overall number of large animals, both male and female, is wearing on the staff that has to lift them on and off the table and in and out of cages. They also exact a toll if they are uncooperative and it is necessary to wrestle with them to accomplish exams and induction. Consider limiting the overall number of large canines, 40 lb (18 kg) and over, to six per day.

CALCULATIONS

Calculating How Many Surgeries Can Be Done in a Day

To calculate the number of patients that can be operated on in a day, use the following formula:

$$\frac{\text{Available surgery minutes}}{\left(\text{Average surgery time } + \text{ Average exam time}\right)} = \frac{\text{Number of surgeries}}{\text{Day}}$$

For example, if your average surgery time is 15 minutes and your average exam time is 5 minutes:

$$\frac{450 \text{ available surgery minutes}}{(15 \text{ minutes average surgery time } + 5 \text{ minutes average exam time})} = \frac{22.5 \text{ surgeries}}{8\text{-hour day}}$$

If you are not doing exams:

$$\frac{450 \text{ available surgery minutes}}{15 \text{ minutes average surgery time}} = \frac{30 \text{ surgeries}}{8\text{-hour day}}$$

Calculating What an Average Surgery Time Needs to Be to Complete a Given Number of Surgeries in a Day

If you know how many surgeries you want to do in a day, you can calculate what your average surgery time needs to be to achieve that goal. Subtract the total minutes you will be spending on exams from your available surgery minutes. For example, if you want to do 30 surgeries and you average 5 minutes per exam, 5 minutes × 30 surgeries equals 150 minutes. Thus, 450 available surgery minutes minus 150 minutes spent on exams equals 300 available surgery minutes.

$$\frac{(\text{Available surgery minutes } - \text{ minutes spent on exams})}{\text{\# of surgeries desired}} = \frac{\text{Average surgery time}}{\text{patient}}$$

For example, if you want to do 30 surgeries in an 8-hour day, and you spend 150 minutes on exams, you need to do an average (medium) surgery in 10 minutes.

$$\frac{450 \text{ available surgery minutes } - 150 \text{ minutes spent on exams}}{30 \text{ surgeries}} = \frac{10 \text{ minutes average surgery time}}{\text{patient}}$$

If the licensed tech does exams, you have more time per surgery.

$$\frac{450 \text{ available surgery minutes}}{30 \text{ desired surgeries}} = \frac{15 \text{ minutes average surgery time}}{\text{patient}}$$

A PROPOSED NEW WAY OF SCHEDULING

Why It Is Needed

When scheduling 30 appointments for a high-volume spay/neuter day, if the day is going to be productive, there have to be some guidelines. This proposed scheduling system recognizes and attempts to take into consideration the variation in the time it takes to do various sterilization surgeries. It addresses a problem long inherent in scheduling in high-volume spay/neuter programs. That problem is that simple numbers do not tell the whole story when setting limits for a scheduled caseload. Thirty large canine spays are not equivalent to 30 feline neuters, etc. This system assigns an equivalency number to each of the surgery types seen in a high-volume spay/neuter practice. The equivalency numbers are based on the time it takes to do each surgery type relative to the time it takes to do an average (medium) surgery.

Relative Surgery Times

Surgery times for various types of surgeries will vary according to the expertise of the doctor and staff and the type of induction used. However, the relative time needed to do a particular type of surgery as compared to doing another type is usually fairly consistent. For example, a large canine spay takes approximately twice as long to do as a small canine spay, and an autoligation feline spay takes half as much time as a small canine spay. For purposes of discussion, I have divided the types of surgeries seen into classes of long, medium, short, and mini, based on the time required to prep them and complete the surgery. Based on the time it takes to do each class of surgery, it can be assigned an equivalency number that reflects how it relates to the average surgery time. This is not an exact system. There are many, many variables influencing surgery times. This system of classification is merely this author's attempt to establish a somewhat common ground for discussion and a means of making the scheduling protocol more relevant. The classification system and concurrent equivalency numbers are listed in Table 3.1.

TABLE 3.1 ■ Equivalency Numbers

Equivalency #	Surgery Class	Surgery type	Sample Time[a]
0.33	Mini	Feline neuters Canine scrotal (puppy) neuters	3 minutes
0.5	Short	Feline autoligation spays Canine prescrotal neuters Canine inguinal cryptorchid neuters	5 minutes
1	Medium (average)	Small canine spays (less than 40 lb, 18 kg) Standard technique feline spays	10 minutes
2	Long	Large canine spays (40 lb, 18 kg or more) Abdominal cryptorchid neuters (canine and feline) Feral cat standard spays, if boxed down	20 minutes

[a]Times listed are this author's average times. Your times may vary, but the times relative to one another should be somewhat consistent.

Equivalency Number Based Scheduling Protocol

- Assign Equivalency numbers
  When scheduling, each appointment is assigned an equivalency number based on the above table. (Table 3.1)
- Keep a Running Total
  When the equivalency numbers add up to thirty (or whatever number of patients you determine is your limit) the caseload for the day has reached its limit. Keeping track of the running total of equivalency points and when they have reached capacity has to be the responsibility of those making the appointments.
- Factor in "No Show" Rates
  If you have a high no-show rate take that into consideration and extend your limits. Surgeries scheduled to allow for no shows should be from the short and mini classifications so that if they do show up the day is not overloaded. For example, once your daily limit of equivalencies has been reached, short and mini surgeries can be added up to a number you have predetermined based on your no-show rate.

A Simplified Scheduling Protocol

Scheduling patients based on equivalency numbers is the most accurate way I have found to ensure a well-balanced surgery schedule. However, it can be rather cumbersome. A somewhat *less accurate* but more easily implemented protocol, based on the principles outlined earlier, is as follows:

- Establish the maximum number of surgeries and maximum number of large dogs to be scheduled.
- Count every large canine *spay* as two surgeries.

In other words, for every large canine *spay* that is scheduled, the maximum number of surgeries goes down by one.

- For example, if your maximum number of surgeries is 30 and you schedule one large canine spay, your new maximum is twenty-nine. If you schedule five large canine spays, your new maximum is twenty-five, and so on.

CHAPTER 4

Setting Up the Surgical Suite

Victoria Valdez, DVM

In general, the goal is to set up the surgical suite for maximum efficiency. Everything you need should be within arm's reach, and the set-up should minimize the number of steps you need to take. (This is true for all workstations including the prep area, the recovery area, the area used for processing packs and instruments, etc.).

SUPPLIES NEEDED FOR SURGERY SET-UP

This is an example only; use surfaces you have available and modify the set-up to your own needs, preserving the principle that for efficiency you need to minimize the amount of reaching and moving you do.

The Surgery Table Area

- A Mayo stand is placed at the end of the surgery table on the surgeon's dominant side.
- A trash can is placed under the Mayo stand.
- A parts bucket is placed under the surgery table or hung from a Mayo stand.
- A high-quality standing mat is placed where the surgeon will be standing.

The Side of the Surgeon (Fig. 4.1)

A shelf, cabinet top, utility cart, or another Mayo stand or combination thereof is used for:

- Gloves
- Space for opening your gloves
- Space for a sterile field (A wrapper from the first pair of gloves or the inner wrapper from the first pack can be used to establish this.)
- Surgical packs
- Drape packs, if packed separately
- Suture on a reel (if desired)
- A sharps container

Behind the Surgeon

A shelf, window ledge, table, etc. is used for:

- Suture packs
- Blades
- Surgical glue
- Tattoo ink (if desired)

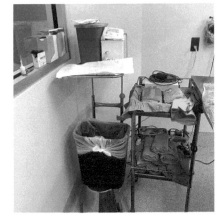

Fig. 4.1 Supplies to The Side and Behind the Surgeon.

OTHER CONSIDERATIONS

One Table vs. Two Tables

In theory, one advantage of using two tables is that there is no lag time between surgeries caused by switching patients. As soon as one surgery is completed, the surgeon moves to the second table. While the surgeon is doing that surgery, the previous patient is removed from the first table and a new one takes its place, and so on, one patient after another. In reality, however, as long as one person is removing the patient and a different person is simultaneously replacing it, the lag time created when switching patients is cancelled out by the time required to move from one table to another. This is especially true if the second table is in a second room.

However, another advantage to having two tables is more valid; that is, it eliminates lag time for the prep person. Once an animal is prepped, it can go on the second surgery table even if the surgeon is not done with the previous surgery and the next animal can be induced and prepped without any lag time.

If two tables are being used, each table must have its own anesthetic machine. This seems obvious, but some individuals have tried moving a portable anesthetic machine from one table to the other. This is cumbersome, dangerous for the patients, and defeats the purpose of using two tables to save time.

Two-Table Configurations (Fig. 4.2)

The two tables can be parallel to one another, at right angles or in a line. They can be free standing with room around them so that the surgeon can work from either side or, as is often the case in mobile clinics, one long side of the table can be against the wall so that, by necessity, the surgeon must work from the side that is away from the wall. Which configuration the surgeon prefers and at which side(s) of the table(s) he or she stands determines how supplies will be set up. The supplies needed are the same as with one table. They are set up to meet the surgeon's needs, keeping in mind that the closer they are to the surgeon, the more efficient. The goal is to keep the amount of reaching necessary and the number of steps taken to a minimum.

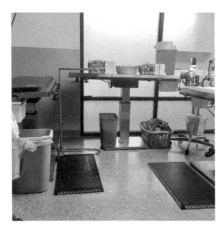

Fig. 4.2   A Sample 2-table Configuration.

Where the Surgeon Stands

Many surgeons use one side of the table for doing spays and the other side for doing neuters. This necessitates either setting up supplies on both sides of the table(s) or taking more steps than are necessary. If this is your normal protocol, consider learning to do neuters on the same side of the table as that from which you do spays. Although it will feel awkward at first, it will soon become routine, and it will save both setup and surgery time as well as the amount of set-up equipment you need, i.e., it is more efficient. If you do not feel comfortable doing neuters on the same side of the table as you do spays, just keep in mind you will sacrifice some efficiency.

SURGERY PACKS

Number and Type of Instruments

Maintaining surgery packs when doing 30 or more surgeries a day is expensive and labor intensive. If at all possible, it is best to use a minimum of instruments per pack (Fig 4.3).

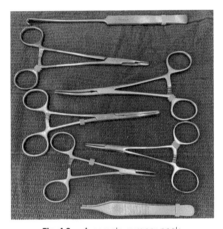

Fig. 4.3   A sample surgery pack.

I am able to do a routine spay or neuter on any size dog or cat with the following instruments.
- A spay hook
- A pair of Olsen-Hager needle holders
- Two carmalts, straight or curved (I prefer straight so I can use extras for feral cat ear tips.)
- Two mosquito forceps, straight or curved (I prefer curved so I can use extras for doing cat neuters.)
- One rat-toothed (or your preference type) thumb forceps

Clamps

Since the number of clamps in the pack is limited for efficiency's sake, carmalts are chosen over kellys or criles because they are needed for large-and giant-breed dog spays, and mosquito forceps are chosen over kellys or criles because they are needed for those tiny kitten spays. Although the number of clamps is limited, it is always possible to open another pack if needed.

Scissors

Scissors are not included in the pack because in most cases the scissors on the Olsen-Hagers or a surgical blade will suffice. Individually packaged and sterilized Mayo or Metzenbaum scissors should be available for those times when they are needed.

"Extra" Instruments

A sterile field is established using the inside wrap from the first surgery pack. As the surgeries progress, unused clamps are placed on the sterile field for use for feral cat ear tips, cat neuters, or for whenever extra clamps are needed. When neuters are performed, the spay hook is not used. It should be saved on the sterile field in case a spay hook is dropped and another needed or there is not one in a pack. Note: Sterile gauze from each pack can be saved in this same manner to be used on subsequent surgeries should the need arise.

ERGONOMICS

A study of ergonomics is beyond the scope of this book. I merely offer these asides regarding things I have personally found helpful in this regard.

Consider Wearing a Lifting Belt

Veterinary medicine is notoriously hard on a person's back. You can lift with your knees and do everything right, but when that patient suddenly jerks and pulls you sidewise, it wrenches your back. Repeated episodes like this take their toll over time. I find my back feels better at the end of the day if I wear a lifting belt (of the type sold at home improvement stores) while I am doing surgery.

Patient Placement

Place the lateral edge of the patient along the edge of the table closest to the surgeon. This helps preclude the back strain created when the surgeon has to lean over the table to reach the patient's midline.

Type of Surgery Table

Uncranking and adjusting the surgery height every time the patient's size changes is cumbersome and hard on the back. Tables that do not have a manual crank locking mechanism for adjusting the table height are preferable to those that do.

Use a High-Quality Extreme Standing Mat

High-volume spay/neuter requires the surgeon to stand on his or her feet for long periods of time. This necessitates a very high-quality standing mat. Extreme standing mats designed to be used on shooting ranges provide excellent cushioning.

Take a Lunch Break

Even if it is not mandated by your state, you and your staff need a lunch break. For efficiency's sake, you are standing in one place and not moving around much. You need to take a break and move around and rest your back. You need to refuel and rehydrate. The afternoon will go a lot smoother if you take a break midday.

CHAPTER 5

Working as a Team

Victoria Valdez, DVM

The only way 30 sterilization surgeries can be performed in a day is with a well-organized team. No one person is more important than another. It is like a well-choreographed dance team. As one dancer performs certain steps, the others are performing theirs so that the overall motion is synchronized to achieve a common effect.

There are many ways to organize the team and what position each member plays. How you organize your team will depend on how many players you have available, your facility, your equipment, and your induction protocol. I offer here one example of what I find most efficient. If you have a system that works for you, by all means stick with it.

In general, I recommend staffing with some variation of the following: Administration staff and at least one each of the following: a licensed technician/anesthetic nurse, a prep person and a recovery person. In general, with the exception of the things only the licensed technician can do, all personnel should be trained to fill all positions. This allows for flexibility in scheduling and covering in the event someone calls in sick or is on vacation, etc. The following is a discussion of the duties and responsibilities of each of these positions, followed by examples of how these duties would play out at various times through the day.

THE TEAM

Administrative Staff

Sufficient staff must be available to schedule appointments, check patients in and out, and process all the computer work and paperwork involved in doing this.

Licensed Technician/Anesthetic Nurse

In many states, anesthesia may be administered only by a licensed or registered veterinary technician or nurse. Whatever designation they are given in your state, be sure you know the law and what duties they can and cannot perform. Adhere to all laws in your state. A licensed technician/anesthetic nurse is an invaluable member of your staff. It is best to have more than one available on any given day. Should he or she not be able to work, you then have backup. Otherwise, in some states, the only other person who can legally administer anesthesia is the doctor. Having the doctor giving anesthesia will greatly diminish a day's production.

Prep Person

It is best to have a designated person to assist the licensed technician/anesthesia nurse with anesthesia. This same person can also prep the patients while the induction nurse is maintaining charts and drawing up drugs for the next patient.

Recovery Person

With 30 patients coming off the table one after the other (this can be as fast as every 3 to 4 minutes with feline neuters), there are often multiple patients in recovery at once, hence the need for at least one designated person in recovery. This is a critical position because when anesthetic deaths occur, it is often during recovery.

The Doctor/Surgeon

From a standpoint of efficiency, it is best if the doctor does what only the doctor can do, i.e., surgery. However, the doctor must be flexible. If, as the doctor is finishing a surgery, the support staff is still busy getting the next patient induced and prepped, the doctor should open his or her own pack, etc. Waiting for staff to do this while the doctor is doing nothing is counterproductive. Whoever has the most time should be performing these duties.

SYNERGY BETWEEN DOCTOR AND STAFF

Support Staff

The support staff makes the surgeon's job easier in countless ways. In fact, the surgeon could not perform his or her job without them. If the surgeon, in turn, makes the jobs of the support staff easier, the more time they will have to aid the surgeon and the more efficient the whole operation will be; i.e., a greater number of surgeries can be performed.

Doctor/Surgeon

There are many things the surgeon can do to make the staff's job easier. It is a synergistic relationship; the more time the surgeon saves his or her staff, the more time the staff will have to perform those duties that directly aid the surgeon. It takes virtually no time away from surgery to be organized in a way that benefits the entire team. For example, the surgeon should consider routinely doing the following:

- Separate instruments.

  Separate clean instruments from dirty instruments. (This pretty much happens automatically while the surgery is performed. The surgeon should keep them that way.) Establish a receptacle with water for used bloody instruments (to make them easier to clean) and a dry receptacle for used clean instruments. That way, your staff does not waste time cleaning clean instruments or, at the very least, sorting through them to determine which are clean and which are dirty.

- Keep drapes and wraps as clean as possible.

  Once instruments are bloody, do not place them back on the pack. Rest them on the drape, which probably already has blood on it, instead of soiling the wrap from the pack.

- Soak bloody drapes.

  Place bloody drapes in a container of cold water. This will remove the blood and keep them looking professional longer.

- Separate clean linens from dirty linens.

  Place clean wraps and drapes in a separate container. Keeping clean linens and dirty linens separate cuts down on man-hours used to do laundry.

- Be self-sufficient.

  Learn to open packages in a sterile manner. You can learn to open blade and suture packages, etc., sterilely on your own. If you forget to open your blade or suture or you need extra gauze, open it yourself. If your team has to stop and help you, there will be a delay in getting your next patient on the table. Following the steps outlined in Figs. 5.1 through 5.5, it is possible to open a package without breaking sterility.

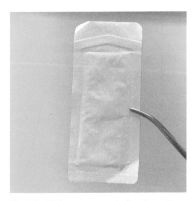

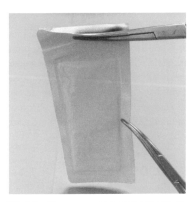

Fig. 5.1 Using a spare sterile clamp from your pack or an "extras pack," grasp the package away from the opening flaps and lock the clamp.

Fig. 5.2 Place a second clamp longitudinally along one of the opening flaps and lock that clamp.

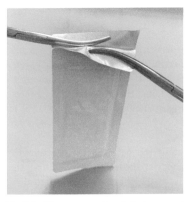

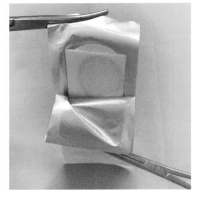

Fig. 5.3 Now remove the first clamp and reposition it longitudinally along the other opening flap and lock it.

Fig. 5.4 Open the flaps by pulling the two opening flaps away from each other.

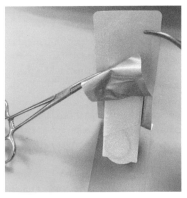

Fig. 5.5 Pour the contents of the package you are opening onto your surgery pack.

- Make use of an "extras pack".
  Open a pack prior to surgery to serve as an "extras pack" from which you can retrieve a duplicate instrument should you drop one or need an extra. This pack can also be used as a sterile field where you can deposit gauze or instruments that you have not used, for use in the next surgery. For example, if you are doing a spay, and you have a cat neuter coming up, and you have used all the appropriate clamps from your "extras pack," you can save a clamp from your spay pack by putting it on your sterile field and then using it to do the upcoming cat neuter. Likewise, if you need more sterile gauze, you have what you need without interrupting your staff.

INDIVIDUAL DUTIES

The following is one example of how to set up the working day with regard to individual responsibilities. There are many ways to do this. This is only one example. Ideally (with the exception of the duties limited by law to only licensed individuals), each member of the staff should be trained to perform the duties of all positions. This allows for flexibility in scheduling staff and provides a method for covering positions in the event someone is sick or on vacation.

Morning Check-in Duties

- Administrative Staff
  The administrative staff has owners fill out paperwork, ask if the patient has any vomiting or diarrhea, when the patient last ate, if vaccines are current, etc. Staff should be trained to answer most questions owners have. If the owner asks about a serious medical problem the patient is currently experiencing, the owner should be referred to a full-service hospital and the sterilization surgery should be postponed until after the problem is addressed.
- Prep person and Recovery Person
  The prep person and the recovery person admit the patient, get the patient's weight and temperature, and record them on the patient's chart. If they see anything they think the doctor should address, they should note it on the chart and bring it to the doctor's attention.
- Licensed Technician or Doctor
  The licensed technician and/or the doctor examine the patient, administer any premed drugs, and record examination details in the chart.

Midday/Surgery Duties

- Administrative Staff
  The administrative staff inputs charges and prepares discharge packets for patients (including aftercare instructions, emergency information, microchip registration information, vaccine schedules, etc.). They also make calls to owners advising them when their pets are done, how they are doing, and when they can be picked up.
- Licensed Technician
  The licensed technician determines patient flow, administers anesthesia, keeps drug logs, and, under direction of the doctor, maintains patient records. This person may also set up the doctor's pack, blade, and suture as the doctor is finishing the surgery. Then he or she removes the patient from the surgery table when the surgery is done.
- Prep person
  The prep person helps the licensed technician with IV injections and intubation. He or she also preps the patient for surgery and puts the patient on the surgery table as the previous patient is being removed. (You can see how this is like a dance: one person is

removing a patient from the table just as another is putting a new patient on. If the same person takes a patient off the table and puts a new one on, there is lag time between the patients.)

- Recovery Person
  The recovery person monitors the patients' breathing, gum color, and body temperature. He or she administers any vaccines, dewormers, and microchips as needed; monitors recovery; and extubates the patient when appropriate and returns them to their cages when it is safe.
- Surgeon
  The doctor performs all sterilization surgeries and deals with any complications that occur and emergencies that arise.

Afternoon/Postop Duties

- Administrative Staff
  The administrative staff collects payments, processes paperwork, and distributes documents and handouts to owners as they pick up their pets.
- Licensed Technician
  The licensed technician checks patients' surgery site, gum color, cognition, and ability to walk before discharging them. He or she goes over aftercare instructions with owner and relays any special instructions from the doctor.
- Prep person and Recovery Person
  When there are no patients in recovery, the prep person and recovery person clean instruments, launder drapes and process and autoclave packs.
- Surgeon
  The doctor checks all patients to be sure they are doing well before leaving for the day.

CHAPTER 6

Establishing Flow (The Order in Which Patients Are Done)

Victoria Valdez, DVM

Flow is the order in which patients are done. It is usually the licensed technician, with or without input from the surgeon, who determines in what order patients will be done. However, a given facility may already have a protocol in place that determines patient order. For example, a facility may do surgeries on patients based on the order in which they checked in to the facility or based on what time the owners are scheduled to pick them up. These are not the most efficient grounds on which to base patient order.

With good flow, as one surgery is done, the patient is removed from the surgery table and a new one replaces it with no lag time between patients. The best person to facilitate this is the licensed technician. I include a discussion of flow in this volume because, if done right, it is a vital part of saving time in a high-volume spay/neuter practice.

Many factors need to be considered when determining patient order, including the induction method, the patient temperament, the estimated time surgery will take, the estimated preparation time, and the estimated time for any ancillary procedures or add-on surgeries. Each practice will have differing surgery times depending on the protocols and skill of those performing these tasks, but the surgery times relative to one another should be fairly consistent (Table 6.1).

TABLE 6.1 ■ Sample Surgery Times

Surgery Class	Surgery Type	Sample Surgery Time[a]
Mini	Feline neuters Canine scrotal (puppy) neuters	3 min
Short	Feline autoligation spays Canine pre-scrotal neuters Canine inguinal cryptorchid neuters	5 min
Medium (Average)	Small canine spays (less than 40 lb, 18 kg) Standard technique feline spays	10 min
Long	Large canine spays (40 lb, 18 kg or more) Abdominal cryptorchid neuters (canine and feline) Feral cat spays, if boxed down	15–20 min

Note that prep times more or less match surgery times.
[a]Surgery times are measured from the time the patient is placed on the table until the next patient is placed on the table. Times listed are this author's average times. Your times may vary.

Use this table along with the principles outlined later to create an optimal patient order for each day's caseload, keeping in mind the need to be flexible if unforeseen circumstances arise. Surgical complications do occur, patients prove intractable who were not so upon examination, a team member calls in sick, etc. It is impossible to predict every eventuality. Doing your best to maximize efficient flow when these interruptions are not occurring makes them less devastating when they do. Although flow is so integral to efficiency, I find it is a difficult concept to teach, and to learn. If you have a technician who is proficient in this, do all you can to keep him or her. He or she is invaluable and will save you time, money, and your sanity. It is extremely frustrating to feel your day slipping away as you stand doing nothing while you are waiting for your next patient to be put on the table.

PRINCIPLES FOR DETERMINING PATIENT ORDER

Minimize Contamination

Always do owned cats before feral cats, to prevent the spread of upper respiratory disease via contaminated equipment such as induction boxes, oxygen bags, and anesthetic machines.

Be Flexible: Do Not Leave The Surgery Table Empty

For example, if a patient that has been preanesthetized with tiletamine is slowly going down, fill in with a mini-surgery (a feline neuter or scrotal canine neuter) while waiting for the tiletamine-induced patient to go down.

Do Risky Patients First

Patients with compromised airways such as chondrodystrophic breeds should not be done right before lunch or at the end of the day (when recovery time is limited or fewer people are around to monitor their recovery). The same is true for patients in late-term pregnancy, who may have an increased risk of bleeding postoperatively.

Match Preparation Times with Sugery Times Whenever Possible

If the patient on the table has a long surgery, such as a large canine spay, the person doing induction should try to induce the patient with an equivalent preparation time so that as the surgeon is finishing one surgery, the next patient is just ready to go on the table. That way, the surgeon is not waiting for the next patient and the next patient is not being anesthetized longer than it needs to be because it is waiting to go on the table. If no matching preparation time patient is available, the induction person should wait an appropriate amount of time to induce the patient with a shorter preparation time so that the previous patient's surgery and the new patient's preparation completion are synchronized. Fortunately, for most types of surgery we do, the preparation time is very similar to the surgery time; i.e., it takes relatively longer to prepare a long surgery like a canine spay, and it is relatively quick to prepare a feline neuter, which is our fastest surgery. Therefore, doing like surgeries in groups is more efficient than alternating long/short, for example, because the preparation time for one surgery matches that for the next. (Doing like-sized patients in groups is also helpful because the breathing bag and table height do not have to be constantly changed).

FACTORS THAT INCREASE SURGERY TIME

Ancillary Surgeries

Ancillary surgeries such as umbilical hernia repair or dewclaw removal prolong surgery time. These ancillary surgeries also prolong preparation time, since the ancillary surgery sites also need to be prepared. Consequently, these patients end up in a longer class of surgery and need to be treated accordingly.

Difficult or Unpredictable Surgeries

The duration of surgery for abdominal cryptorchids, females in late stages of pregnancy, obese females, or those who have had previous C-sections (and may have extensive adhesions) can be prolonged. Due to this unpredictability it is best not to do these surgeries where time is limited: for example, before a set lunch break time or as the last surgery of the day. To allow for the possibility that the surgery time may be prolonged, these surgeries should be treated as if they are in a longer class of surgery than that in which they would normally fall. Preparation times are not affected, so they remain in their original preparation time classification. This means their preparation time should match the surgery time of the patient ahead of them. The preparation time of the patient that follows them should match their prolonged surgery time.

FACTORS THAT PROLONG *PREPARATION* TIME

A surgery that normally has a short preparation time may actually have a long preparation time if inhalant anesthesia is used for induction, the patient is hard to handle or requires add-on procedures during preparation, or the licensed technician or preparation person is inexperienced. If any of these conditions are present, the patient's classification regarding preparation time should be adjusted to the next longer classification. Since these patients have a prolonged preparation time, they should follow patients that have an equally long surgery time. These factors do not alter surgery time. Consequently, once this patient goes into surgery, the next patient that should be induced is one whose preparation time matches this patient's surgery time.

Inhalant Anesthesia

A complete discussion of the different induction protocols available is beyond the scope of this text. What you use may be determined by your personal preference or may have been predetermined by the facility for which you work. Choices are often made based on safety, availability, ease of application, and control drug status. If the patient is easy to handle, induction by injection is generally faster and safer than inhalant anesthesia via box or mask. When figuring your preparation time, extra time must be added for inhalant induction.

Add-on Procedures During Preparation

Intravenous catheterization, fluid administration, extraction of deciduous teeth, and ear tipping can all prolong preparation time.

Fractious or Feral Patients

These patients often require significantly more time to induce. Safety of those doing the induction is paramount. Transferring feral cats from traps to induction boxes can be critical. Large amounts of time can be lost if the cat gets loose. In my all-feline practice, I found the following protocol useful for those cats that could not be induced via injection through the trap:

- With the cat in the humane trap, a clear trash bag large enough to fit over the trap is placed over the entire trap.
- A large endotracheal tube is inserted into the open end of the bag.
- The end of the bag is gathered around the attachment end of the endotracheal tube and secured with a rubber band and or tape.
- The anesthetic machine is attached to the endotracheal tube and anesthesia administered through it.

■ The downside of this method is that it uses a lot of anesthesia. It also exposes the person doing anesthesia to a large amount of inhalant gas. The upside is that there is little chance the patient will escape, and the handler's safety from teeth or claws is assured as long as the patient is not handled until it is well anesthetized.

Technician Skill and Availability

Obviously, an experienced technician will be faster than a new one. No one is born with these skills. Allowances must be made for learning time, but a new person will almost always increase preparation times until he or she becomes accustomed to your protocols and gains experience. Careful training and patience are investments that will pay off well over time.

IN CONCLUSION

The patient order that works best for you and your practice is not necessarily what works best for me, and what works best one day is not necessarily what works best another day. In general, I prefer to work in order of degree of difficulty, from the most difficult to the least, risky or unpredictable surgeries first, then longest to shortest surgeries. Keeping in mind the earlier principles and consequent exceptions, after risky surgeries, I prefer to do large canine spays first, then any abdominal cryptorchid neuters, then small canine spays, then canine neuters (any size: large to small), then owned cats, then feral cats. During "kitten season," I turn that around and do cats first (owned, then feral) in case any of them are late-term pregnant, thereby allowing more time to watch them postoperatively.

CHAPTER 7

Saving Time in Surgery

Victoria Valdez, DVM

Previous chapters have discussed how time is saved via judicious scheduling, efficient worksta-tion set-up, coordinated teamwork, and good patient flow. This chapter deals with time-saving techniques involving actual surgery. Being proficient in any one of the aforementioned areas is not enough to make high-volume spay/neuter possible. All of these elements must come to-gether in a cohesive whole to produce a successful high-volume spay/neuter program. Below are some surgical techniques I have found time saving. This is by no means a comprehensive list of all time-saving techniques used by all spay/neuter veterinarians. They are merely those that I find to be safe and effective in my hands. My hope is that some or all of them may be helpful to you.

TECHNIQUES THAT ENHANCE SAFETY AND THEREBY SAVE TIME

If there is one thing that saves time in high-volume spay/neuter, it is doing everything as safely as possible, within the parameters with which we work. All techniques that enhance safety SAVE TIME because nothing eats up time like complications. Using safe practices will minimize complications and thereby also increase your time efficiency.

Safely Using The Spay Hook

Care must be taken when using a spay hook. For efficiency, incisions are typically small in high-volume spay/neuter. When the incision is small, it makes it imperative that a spay hook be used to locate and exteriorize the uterine horn. However, care must be taken not to damage the spleen or other internal organs with the spay hook. The index finger is used to locate and assess the position and extent of the spleen. If necessary, the surgeon gently, manually retracts the spleen out of the way. The spay hook is positioned so that the hook points to the right body wall and it is swept down the body wall to the inside fold of the *right* rear leg (the right side is used because the spleen resides primarily, but not always entirely, on the left and is less likely to be in the way on the right side). Then the point of the hook is rotated 360 degrees and swept slightly toward the midline incision. If the uterine horn is engaged, tension will be felt on the hook. Too much tension could indicate that a ureter has been engaged. If so, the hook is disengaged and another attempt is made to engage the uterine horn. When the uterine horn is engaged, it is gently retracted up through the incision.

Making The Incision More Cranially in Canines That Have Given Birth

When performing a canine spay surgery the incision must be placed so that it is possible to exteriorize both the ovaries and the uterine bifurcation. Where the incision is made is dependent on the reproductive status of the patient. This is best accessed based on the size of the patient's nipples. In canines that have not reproduced, the nipples are small. The size of a nipple in a nul-liparous female versus one that has had had puppies is of course relative. This can sometimes be difficult to determine. It is helpful to picture an appropriately sized puppy's mouth nursing on the nipple. If it does not seem like a puppy could get its mouth around the nipple, the patient has probably never nursed puppies.

The reason the location of the incision varies is because the pliability of the uterus varies with the patient's reproductive status. Once the female gives birth, the uterus is stretched out and it is possible to make that more cranial incision. This is significant because when the incision is cranial (just caudal to the umbilicus), it makes it easier to exteriorize the uterus and it is less likely to be necessary to break the suspensory ligament.

In a canine spay, if it is possible to make the abdominal incision just caudal to the umbilicus, which puts the incision closer to the ovaries so that they are easier to access, thereby saving the surgeon time. A more cranial incision increases also increases the ability to exteriorize the ovaries, making related structures more visible and thereby increasing safety.

In nulliparous animals, the uterus is tighter, so to be able to reach both the ovaries *and the uterine bifurcation*, the incision must be further caudal. In these nulliparous patients, the incision is made halfway between the umbilicus and the pubis.

NOTE: In all cats, the abdominal incision is made halfway between the umbilicus and the pubis.

Carefully Breaking The Suspensory Ligament

When performing a spay surgery, it is necessary to elevate the ovaries far enough out of the incision that the surgeon can clearly see what he or she is doing. It is also important to be able to leave enough space between the ovarian ligature and the ovary that the surgeon can easily incise the pedicle far enough below the ovary to ensure that no ovarian tissue is left in the patient. To achieve this, it may be necessary to break or stretch the suspensory ligament. Where possible, it is preferable to not break the ligament because, on rare occasions, breaking it can lead to inadvertent tearing of adjacent vessels inside the pedicle and subsequent bleeding. Making the abdominal incision just cranial to the umbilicus, as is possible in canines who have had a previous pregnancy, makes it less likely to have to break the suspensory ligament. In nulliparous canines, the incision is between the umbilicus and the pubis, and loosening or breaking the suspensory ligament is more likely to be necessary. If it is necessary to loosen or break the suspensory ligament, the surgeon may try using the index finger to apply longitudinal pressure along it. This often will stretch the ligament enough so that it does not need to be broken. If not enough exposure of the ovary is achieved with just stretching the ligament, the surgeon should exert more even, gentle pressure as far cranially on the ligament as possible, until the ligament breaks. Once the ligament is broken, the surgeon checks for bleeding from the pedicle and ligates vessels as needed.

Placing Ligatures Securely

There are many ways to ligate the ovarian arteries and uterine stump. Bleeding from the stump and/or pedicles is the leading cause of death post spay. So, whatever method is used needs to be safe and secure. This author prefers a protocol that combines use of a miller's knot and large-gauge chromic gut. It has proved to be a very safe and efficient combination. A miller's knot is an extremely secure knot. It forms two encircling loops with a bump in between the two "ligatures" that keeps the knot from sliding. Chromic gut is used because it has relatively little memory and therefore stays where it is put. Larger-than-normal gauge suture is used to make it possible to really tighten the knot without breaking the suture. NOTE: The author has found that in most cases with these ligatures, and those used in canine neuters, it is not necessary to strip the pedicle, stump, or cord of fat. Simple manipulation gets rid of the majority of the fat, and then using larger-gauge gut makes it possible to press through the fat with the ligature. This is not true, however, when doing self-ties during cat neuters. In that instance, stripping the fat is recommended so that the fat does not interfere with the seating of the knot.

Placing Ligatures Securely in Large, Obese, in Estrus, or Pregnant Patients

In large, in estrus, or pregnant patients, the blood supply is increased. In obese patients, the vessels are very friable. Therefore, for safety's sake, extra precautions should be taken with ligatures in these patients. An extra clamp is used cranial to the ovary where the ligature will be placed. The miller's knot used on the ovarian pedicles in these patients is modified. A regular miller's knot is placed around the pedicle in the grove made by the clamp with three throws to secure the knot. Then the suture is wrapped around once more and secured with three additional throws. The uterine arteries are ligated prior to ligating the uterine stump. Then a miller's knot encompasses the arterial ligature and the uterus.

Closing Incisions Securely

High-volume spay/neuter patients are often in situations where they are not closely supervised postop. Increased activity may put undue stress on their incision lines. Because of its strength and durability, polydioxanone is preferred for closing incisions in these patients. Another consideration is the use of at least one-size-larger gauge suture than would be used in general practice. Knots are secured with extra throws and tags are left slightly longer and glue is applied to the knots where appropriate.

Providing Thorough Aftercare Instructions

Clear, concise, and thorough take-home instructions (in languages prevalent in your area, if possible) are a necessity for our clientele. Providing good take-home instructions saves time by decreasing the amount of time necessary for follow-up phone calls and rechecks. In some cases, good aftercare instructions could be life-saving.

- Body Temperature and Hygiene
  Owners should be advised of the importance of keeping the patient warm, dry, and clean postop.
- Monitoring Gum Color
  Clients should be shown what normal gum color looks like and advised to monitor it for 24 hours.
- Provide a Hotline Number
  Where available, a number should be given to owners that they can call if they have questions overnight.
- Establish a Relationship With a 24-Hour Hospital
  If possible, protocols should be pre-established with an emergency hospital in your area for problems that require emergency treatment overnight.
- Provide E-Collars for Dogs
  An Elizabethan collar should be sent home with ALL dogs (along with good instructions on how to use it, including using small bowls for feeding with the collar on). Owners should be advised that if the collar is not used, your facility will not be responsible for aftercare if the dog gets at its incision. If they schedule a recheck for a problem postop, advise them they must bring the e-collar with them. A pristine e-collar is a clear indication it was not used.
- Provide Instructions for Body Suits for Cats
  Cats tend to get their paws or jaws caught in an Elizabethan collar, so instead consider sending home instructions on how to make a body suit from a sweatshirt sleeve, a sock, or a baby onesie for cats that are bothering their incisions. Instructions are available online.

■ Keeping the Patient Quiet Postoperatively
Consider instructions for giving diphenhydramine orally to keep overly active dogs quiet postoperatively once the anesthesia has fully worn off. (This may be especially helpful for canine neuters.)

TECHNIQUES THAT SAVE TIME

Tattooing to Prevent Unnecessary Surgery

The time this saves may be your own. Our patients often change owners, sometimes without known sterilization history. In many states, by law, animals cannot be adopted from a shelter without being sterilized. When an animal comes into a shelter, its status regarding sterilization is often unknown. Too often, surgery must be done on an animal who has already been spayed or neutered. This necessitates an abdominal exploration that is far more invasive than the original sterilization surgery. It requires a longer incision, more organ manipulation, and a longer anesthesia time. Besides putting the patient at risk, it is a waste of time and resources, all of which could have been avoided with a simple tattoo.

■ Females
If a female dog or cat was spayed at a young age, a scar may not be noticeable. If a scar is visible, it does not necessarily mean the surgery performed was a spay. (In this instance, it helps to evaluate the nipples. If the nipples are small and the patient has an appropriately placed and sized scar, the evidence is good that she has been spayed, but this is by no means infallible.)

■ Males
Just because a male dog or cat does not have testicles does not mean it has been neutered. It may be a bilateral cryptorchid.

■ Male Dogs
Male dogs often have a natural white line down the median of the prescrotal area that can be mistaken for a scar. Do not use that "scar" as evidence of its having been neutered. (If a scar that shows suture marks is present and the penis is small, that is better evidence for having been neutered.)

■ Male Adult Cats
Male cats lose the spikes on their penises within about 30 days of being neutered. Examination of the penis for the presence or absence of these spikes is a reliable indication of the cat's sterilization status. It may be necessary to anesthetize the patient to do this, however. I do not tattoo adult male cats.

■ Male Kittens
The spikes in male kittens do not develop until about 6 months of age. Since kittens are now commonly neutered as young as 2 months of age, there is a window of time where it is impossible to tell if a kitten without testicles has been neutered or just hasn't developed spikes yet. I tattoo kittens between 2 and 4 months of age.

■ Technique
It is not necessary to make a long tattoo. If green tattoo ink is used, just a dot is enough to alert the observer to the fact that the animal has been sterilized. Using the blunt end of the surgical blade, a dab of tattoo ink is placed at the cranial end of the incision (i.e., the opposite end from where the subcuticular knot is). As the skin is closed with surgical glue, the ink and knot are also covered with glue.
(Author's note: After having done thousands of surgeries involving tattoos, I have not seen an increased incidence of incision dehiscence or infection. However, if you are concerned about this, you can always apply the tattoo to a small shallow skin incision adjacent to the spay or neuter incision).

Maintaining Sterility Between Patients Without Rescrubbing

It is a common practice in high-volume spay/neuter to not rescrub and regown between patients. This is probably the single most time-saving modification we use. However, doing this makes it necessary to take other precautions to enhance sterility.

- Do Not Pre-Open Gloves

  Since reliance on the sterility of the surgical gloves is magnified by not scrubbing between surgeries, gloves should not be opened until the surgeon is ready to start a surgery. The common practice among spay/neuter veterinarians of pre-opening gloves is not recommended.

- Avoid Bare Hands Between Surgeries

  Once the surgeon has scrubbed, gowned, and put on his or her first pair of gloves, his or her hands should not be bare until the last surgery of the session is done. The surgeon leaves his or her gloves on from the previous surgery until he or she changes into the gloves for the current surgery.

- The Surgeon's Gown Should Be Kept Sterile

  Sterile drapes for each surgery should be large enough that they drape over the edge of the surgery table. This prevents the surgeon's gown from becoming contaminated should it touch the edge of the table.

- Rescrub When Necessary

  The surgeon should rescrub and regown after lunch and whenever sterility is broken.

Small Incisions

The smaller the incision, the less time spent closing it. However, if the surgeon is new to high volume, the size of the incision should be whatever is comfortable. For efficiency's sake, the incision for a spay does not need to be much bigger than the size of the patient's ovary, including any surrounding fat and connective tissue. For this author, for an uncomplicated spay, that tends to be about 1.5 inches (3. cm) in large dogs 40 lb (18 kg) and up and about ¾ in (1.9 cm) in small dogs and cats. In general, the more proficient the surgeon becomes, the smaller his or her incisions will become. However, the surgeon should never hesitate to enlarge the incision as needed. The surgeon should never try to force the ovary through too small an incision. It is common to need to extend the incision if there is excessive fat around the ovary, the ovary is cystic or for any other reason enlarged, the patient is pregnant, or the tissues are friable as in the obese or postpartum patient. The surgeon should always make the incision long enough to see and do what is needed comfortably.

No Skin Sutures

It is possible to securely appose the skin using a combination of a subcuticular suture pattern and surgical glue. This negates the need for skin sutures, which in turn negates the need for rechecks for suture removal. Eliminating skin suture placement and suture removal appointments saves considerable time from the surgeon's day. Polydioxanone suture is used for strength and longevity. To compensate for the fact that there are no skin sutures, consider using one-size-larger gauge suture for greater strength in both abdominal and subcuticular closures.

Surgical Protocols

CHAPTER 8

Small Canine Spay

Victoria Valdez, DVM

Presented here is the protocol I use for a small canine spay (less than 40 lb, 18 kg). It has been developed over many years of doing exclusively high-volume spay/neuter. Each time I modified or refined my technique, it was with the goal of making it either safer or more time efficient. This protocol works for me, but what protocol you use is a matter of personal preference. Even if you are happy with your current protocol, there may be elements of what I describe here that are new to you and sound like something that you might want to try. Keep in mind that to incorporate something new into your regimen, you must do it at least 10–20 times before it feels comfortable.

PROTOCOL

Make the Abdominal Incisions

A ventral midline incision is made in the skin just caudal to the umbilicus in primiparous or multiparous females and halfway between the umbilicus and the pubis in nulliparous females. Goal incision sizes are 0.75 in (1.9 cm) to 1.5 in (3.8 cm) depending on the size of the animal.

The patient shown in Fig. 8.1 is nulliparous (note the small nipples).

Blunt dissection is used to reach the abdominal wall. An incision is then made through the linea alba (Fig. 8.2).

For both incisions, the blade is held with the sharp surface pointing up, to avoid incising abdominal organs.

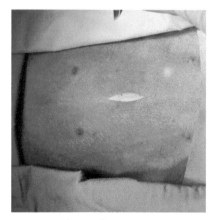

Fig. 8.1 Skin incision.

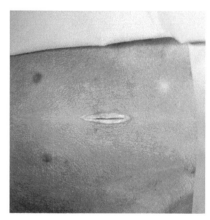

Fig. 8.2 Incision in linea alba.

Exteriorize the Right Uterine Horn

The right uterine horn is retrieved by sweeping the spay hook inside the right abdominal wall to the inside fold of the *right* back leg. Care is taken to avoid the spleen (Fig. 8.3).

The spay hook is then pulled cranially toward the incision to engage the uterine horn. Once the right horn is engaged, it is passed through the incision (Fig. 8.4).

The horn is then followed manually to the right ovary (Fig. 8.5).

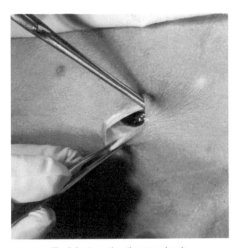

Fig. 8.3   Inserting the spay hook.

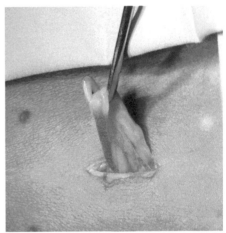

Fig. 8.4   Exteriorize the horn.

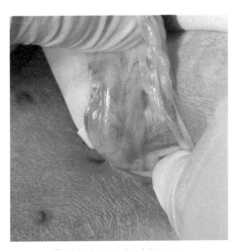

Fig. 8.5   Locate the right ovary.

Ready the Right Ovarian Pedicle for Ligation

The surgeon's index finger is used to make a window in the mesovarium, adjacent to the proper ligament. It is not necessary to extend the window cranially along the ovarian pedicle; it will automatically stretch to do this. This window is necessary for a ligature to be placed around the ovarian pedicle (Fig. 8.6).

A clamp is placed on the proper ligament of the right ovary (Fig. 8.7). Only one clamp is used for greater visualization and ease of operation. (NOTE: A new surgeon may prefer to use multiple clamps until he or she is comfortable doing spays. The surgeon should do what feels most secure.)

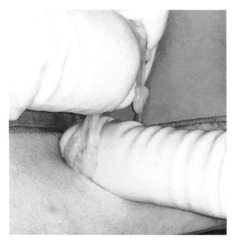

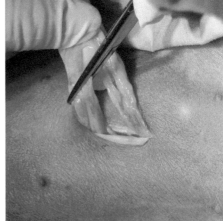

Fig. 8.6 Make a window in the mesovarium.   **Fig. 8.7** Clamp the proper ligament.

Loosen or Break the Suspensory Ligament

If loosening the suspensory ligament is necessary to adequately exteriorize the ovary, gentle longitudinal digital pressure is exerted along the suspensory ligament to achieve this (Fig. 8.8).

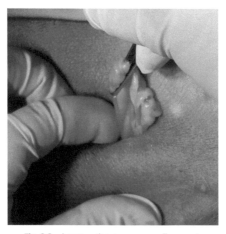

Fig. 8.8 Loosen the suspensory ligament.

Ligate the Ovarian Pedicle with a Miller's Knot

Once the ovary is exposed well enough for good visualization, the right ovarian pedicle is ligated using a Miller's knot. A Miller's knot is utilized for increased knot security. It, in effect, forms two ligatures with a bump between them that minimizes slipping. Chromic gut is used because it has relatively little memory and therefore is less likely than some newer suture materials to come untied. Another advantage of chromic gut is that it requires only three throws on each knot. Because the surgeon needs to be able to really tighten the knots without the suture breaking, larger-than-normal gauge suture (2-0 chromic gut in small dogs) is used. The following are directions for tying a Miller's knot.

- Make a Loop in the Suture
  Using an approximate 16–18 inches of suture, a 4-inch loop is made in one end of the suture. The loop is placed on the far side of the part requiring ligation (Fig. 8.9).
- Place One Tail Through the Loop
  One tail of the suture is placed through the loop and grasped with needle holders (Fig. 8.10).
- Place the Suture
  The suture is slid to the desired location below the ovary. Because of adherent fat and connective tissue, the ovary is not always visible. However, its location can be determined by palpation. A minimum of a clear quarter inch (6 mm), preferably more, is left between the ovary and the ligature, so that the pedicle can be cleanly transected. Leaving even a small amount of ovarian tissue in the patient can lead to ovarian cysts, persistent estrus, and stump pyometra (Fig. 8.11).
- Tighten the First Ligature
  Pulling the two tails of the suture in opposite directions secures the first of the two ligatures formed by one Miller's knot (Fig. 8.12).
- Adjust Placement for Second Ligature
  The tails of the suture are placed up in a V formation to aid in forming the bump between the two ligatures of the knot, prior to tying the second ligature (Fig. 8.13).
- Tie Second Ligature
  The second ligature is tied, leaving space between it and the first ligature, so that a bump is formed between the two (Fig. 8.14).
- Secure With Three Throws
  The knot is completed with three throws, and the sutures are clipped (Fig. 8.15).

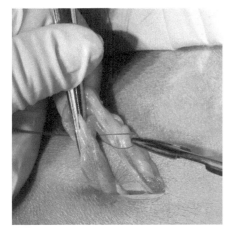

Fig. 8.9 Making a loop.

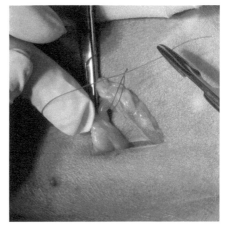

Fig. 8.10 Tail through the loop.

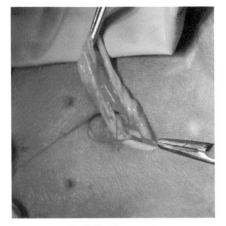

Fig. 8.11 Placement.

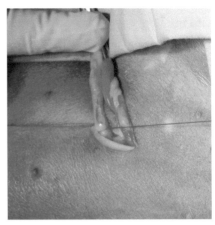

Fig. 8.12 First ligature.

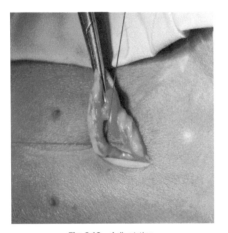

Fig. 8.13 Adjust ties.

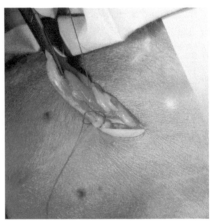

Fig. 8.14 Second ligature.

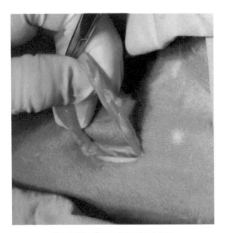

Fig. 8.15 Complete the knot.

Transect the Pedicle Cranial to the Ovary

The ovarian pedicle is transected, leaving a minimum of 1/8-inch tag on the ovarian pedicle cranial to the ovary (Fig. 8.16).

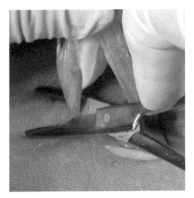

Fig. 8.16   Transect the pedicle.

Detach the Mesometrium from the Uterus

Locate the uterine artery lateral to the uterine horn (Fig. 8.17).

The surgeon's index finger is used to create a window in the mesometrium lateral to the artery (Fig. 8.18).

That window is extended laterally across the margin of the mesometrium portion of the broad ligament, and the mesometrium is detached from the uterus lateral to the uterine artery to the level of the uterine body (Fig. 8.19).

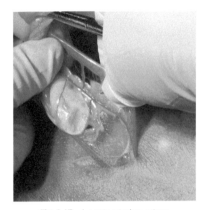

Fig. 8.17   Locate uterine artery.

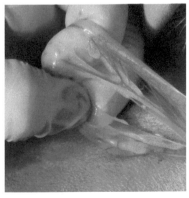

Fig. 8.18   Make a window.

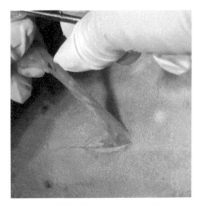

Fig. 8.19   Detach mesometrium.

Locate and Ligate the Left Ovary/Exteriorize the Uterus

The left horn is followed from the bifurcation to the left ovary and the previous steps are repeated for the left ovary and mesometrium. The uterine horns, with both ovaries attached, are exteriorized (Fig. 8.20).

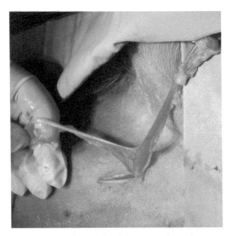

Fig. 8.20 Exteriorized uterus and ovaries.

Ligate the Uterus

The uterus is ligated using a Miller's knot of 2-0 chromic gut, between the bifurcation and the cervix (Fig. 8.21).

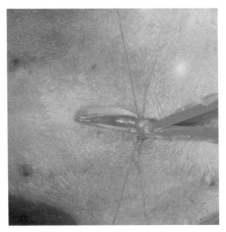

Fig. 8.21 Ligate the uterus with a Miller's knot.

Transect the Uterus

Once the ligature is secure, the uterus is transected cranial to the ligature, and the ovaries and uterus are removed, thus completing the ovariohysterectomy portion of the surgery (Fig. 8.22).

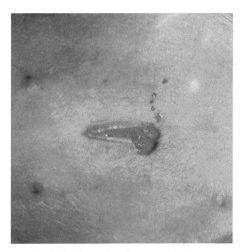

Fig. 8.22 Transect and remove the uterus.

Close the Linea Alba with a Cruciate Suture

The linea is closed using a cruciate suture. NOTE: If your incision is longer than 0.75 in, refer to Chapter 9, Large Canine Spay, for instructions on how to do a continuous cruciate pattern. The cruciate suture starts and stops in the same place, making it possible to have just one knot. Because that one knot must therefore be extremely secure, two extra throws are added to the knot (for a total of six throws) and the suture ends are left long (a little less than one eighth inch). For strength and durability, polydioxanone suture is used. Anticipating that the patient is likely to be more active postoperatively than is desirable, suture one size larger than is normally used in general practice is utilized. For small dogs this is 2-0 polydioxanone.

- First Bite
  A full-thickness bite is taken in the caudal end of the incision. The bite begins in the linea on the far side from the surgeon and passes full thickness through the linea. The needle is then is passed across the incision, up through the linea on the side of the incision nearest the surgeon (Fig. 8.23).
- Second Bite
  A second identical bite is taken at the cranial end of the incision (Fig. 8.24). This forms a half cruciate (Fig. 8.25).
- Form Complete Cruciate
  The two ends of the suture are tied together to form the complete cruciate (Fig. 8.26).
- Apply Six Throws
  Since this pattern does not have a knot at the beginning, it acts like a purse string if pulled tight. For that reason, the ends are not pulled tight until after the third throw. Six throws are applied for security (Fig. 8.27).
- Leave the Tags Long
  For extra security, the tags on the knot are left approximately 1/8-inch long (Fig. 8.28).

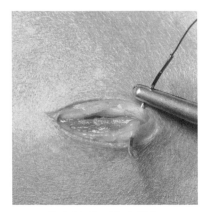

Fig. 8.23 Cruciate first bite.

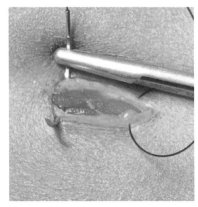

Fig. 8.24 Cruciate second bite.

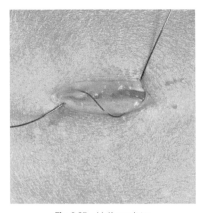

Fig. 8.25 Half cruciate.

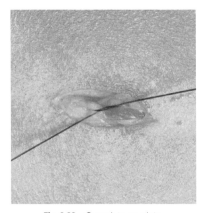

Fig. 8.26 Complete cruciate.

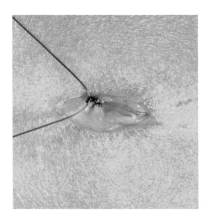

Fig. 8.27 Six throws.

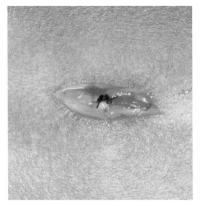

Fig. 8.28 Long tags.

Close the Skin with a Subcuticular Mattress Suture

The subcuticular tissue is closed with polydioxanone with a subcuticular mattress suture with one knot.

- First Bite
  The first bite starts deep at the caudal end of the incision, on the side nearest the surgeon, and comes up just under the skin at the cranial end of the incision (Fig. 8.29).
- Second Bite
  The needle is moved to the opposite side of the incision and a subcuticular bite is taken in a cranial to caudal direction (Fig. 8.30).
- The Knot
  Since this suture has only one knot, it will gather up like a purse string if it is tightened too soon. The suture is not pulled tight until after the third throw is placed. One extra throw is added to this knot (for a total of five throws) (Fig. 8.31).
- The Suture Ends
  The suture ends are cut off even with the knot. If any more throws are added or the ends are left long, the knot will not bury properly (Fig. 8.32).

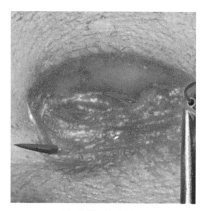

Fig. 8.29 First bite.

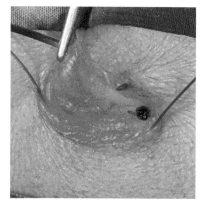

Fig. 8.30 Second bite.

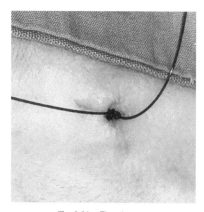

Fig. 8.31 Five throws.

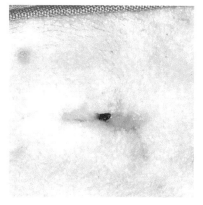

Fig. 8.32 Ends short.

Consider Applying a Tattoo

Tattooing the patient helps to prevent an unnecessary abdominal exploratory in the future and the inherent risks associated with it.

- Apply the Ink
  Using the blunt end of the surgical blade, a dab of tattoo ink is placed at the cranial end of the incision (Fig. 8.33).

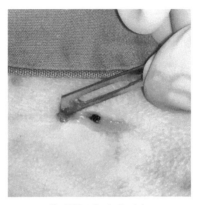

Fig. 8.33   Apply the ink.

Apply Tissue Glue to the Skin

- Apply the Glue
  Tissue glue is applied to the skin being careful to cover the tattoo ink so that it will not get all over the owner's car, clothes, and furniture. For extra safety, a drop of glue is placed on the subcuticular suture's knot to make it more secure (Fig. 8.34).
- Pinch and Hold
  The skin edges are apposed and held together a few seconds to allow the glue to dry (Fig. 8.35).
- Finished Closure
  The finished closure is a small incision with an even smaller tattoo. A larger tattoo is not necessary because any ink at all is enough to alert the viewer to the fact that this animal has been sterilized (Fig. 8.36).

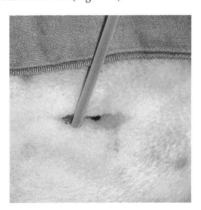

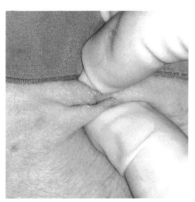

Fig. 8.34   Apply the glue.   **Fig. 8.35**   Pinch and hold.

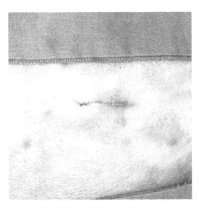

Fig. 8.36 Finished closure.

OTHER CONSIDERATIONS

Pregnancy, Obesity, or Estrus

If the patient is late-term pregnant, very obese, or in estrus, refer to the Large Canine Spay Protocol.

Lactation

When milk is present in the mammary glands, care must be taken to avoid incising the mammary tissue. If the glands are incised, milk will leak into the incision. This will delay healing and could lead to infection or dehiscence.

TROUBLESHOOTING

The Ligature on the Ovarian Pedicle is too Close to the Ovary

- Incise the Connective Tissue
  While traction is simultaneously applied to the ovary, one side of the connective tissue overlying the caudal pole of the ovary is carefully incised (care is taken not to incise the ovary).
- Create Space
  The traction mentioned earlier will cause the connective tissue to peel away from the ovary. More space will thereby be created between the ovary and the ligature.
- Transect the Connective Tissue
  The connective tissue is then transected, leaving a minimum of a 1/8-inch tag on the pedicle above the ligature.

The Knot of the Subcuticular Suture will not Bury

- Cut Only the Nonneedle End of the Subcuticular Suture
  If the knot of the subcuticular suture is not going to bury, this should be evident prior to the surgeon cutting the suture ends. If this is the case, only the nonneedle end of the suture should be cut initially (Fig. 8.37).

- Take the Needle "Deep"

  A bite is taken with the needle through the incision into the subcutaneous tissue and brought back to the surface (Fig. 8.38).

  NOTE: If this technique is used on a pre-scrotal neuter, the bite should be made away from but just parallel to the midline to avoid the urethra.

- Overretract the Suture

  The suture is then pulled tight (overretracted) and then cut off at the skin. This should bury the knot (Fig. 8.39).

  Once the knot is buried, the tattoo and glue are applied, and the skin is apposed as described above.

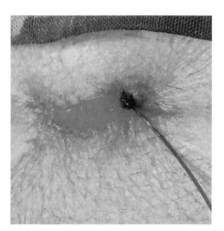

Fig. 8.37 Cut one end.

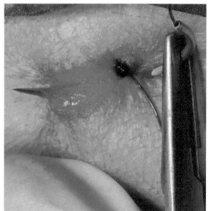

Fig. 8.38 Deep bite.

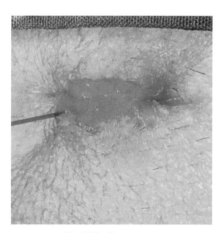

Fig. 8.39 Overretract.

CHAPTER 9

Large Canine Spay

Victoria Valdez, DVM

A large canine spay differs enough from a small canine spay that it deserves its own chapter. Large canines have a more intense blood supply and are often overweight. I have not found an easy way to do a large canine spay. The best way to save time on this surgery is to take all the time you need to do everything you can to avoid complications or having to redo anything. The following protocol is often appropriate for dogs over 40 lb (18 kg), late-term pregnant animals, and in heat and obese dogs of any size. It is really not about the size of the patient but rather the size of the blood vessels and how much fat is present.

If the vessels are large or engorged or there is a large amount of fat present (which causes the vessels to be very friable), the large canine protocol is indicated. For example, the small canine protocol may work well on a young, lean dog weighing 60 lb and conversely it may be necessary to use the large canine protocol on a 20-lb canine who is in the final weeks of pregnancy.

Make The Abdominal Incisions

A ventral midline incision is made in the skin just caudal to the umbilicus in primaparous or multiparous females and halfway between the umbilicus and the pubis in nulliparous females.

Note the large nipples in this multiparous female (Fig. 9.1).

The incision starts just caudal to the umbilicus and the goal incision size is 1.5 in (3.8 cm) (Fig. 9.2).

Blunt dissection is used to reach the linea alba. An incision is then made through the linea alba. For both incisions, the blade is held with the sharp surface pointing up, to avoid incising abdominal organs (Fig. 9.3).

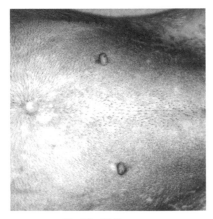

Fig. 9.1 Multiparous.

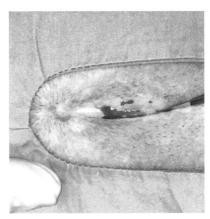

Fig. 9.2 Skin incision.

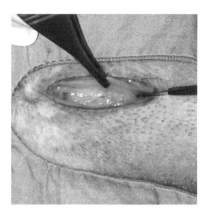

Fig. 9.3 Linea.

Exteriorize The Right Uterine Horn

The right uterine horn is retrieved by sweeping the spay hook inside the right abdominal wall down to the inside fold of the *right* back leg. The right side is used to avoid injuring the spleen. The spay hook is then pulled cranially toward the incision to engage the uterine horn. Once the horn is engaged, it is passed through the incision. The horn is then followed manually to the right ovary.

Ready The Right Ovarian Pedicle for Ligation

The surgeon's index finger is used to make a window in the mesovarium adjacent to the proper ligament. It is not necessary to extend the window cranially along the ovarian pedicle; it will automatically stretch to do this. This window is necessary for a ligature to be placed around the ovarian pedicle (Fig. 9.4).

A clamp is then placed on the proper ligament of the ovary (Fig. 9.5).

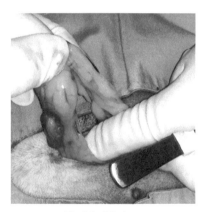

Fig. 9.4 Window.

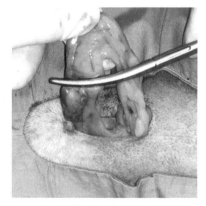

Fig. 9.5 Clamp.

Loosen or Break The Suspensory Ligament

If loosening the suspensory ligament is necessary to adequately exteriorize the ovary, gentle longitudinal digital pressure is exerted along the suspensory ligament to achieve this.

Place a Second Clamp

Once the ovary is exposed enough for good visualization for ligature placement, a second clamp is placed below the ovary in the desired ligature location. The clamp crushes the tissues, creating a trough for the ligature to rest in. It is removed before the ligature is placed (Fig. 9.6).

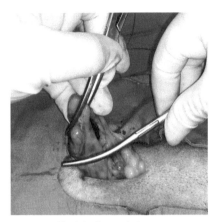

Fig. 9.6   Second clamp.

Ligate The Ovarian Pedicle With a Miller's Knot

A standard Miller's knot forms two ligatures with a bump between them, making it a very secure way to ligate. For large, obese, in estrus, or pregnant dogs, the Miller's knot is modified by the addition of an extra loop around the pedicle, thereby creating three ligatures.

Chromic gut is used for security. Because it has relatively little memory, it is less likely than newer suture materials to come untied. Another advantage of chromic gut is that it requires only three throws on each knot. Because the surgeon needs to be able to really tighten the knots without the suture breaking, larger than normal gauge suture (0 or #1 chromic gut in large dogs) is used.

- Make a Loop in the Suture
  Using an approximate 16–18 in of suture, a 4-in loop is made in one end of the suture. The loop is placed on the far side of the pedicle (Fig. 9.7).
- Place One Tail Through the Loop
  One tail of the suture is placed through the loop and grasped with needle holders (Fig. 9.8).
- Tighten the First Ligature
  Placing the suture in the grove formed by the second clamp and pulling the two tails of the suture in opposite directions secure the first of the two ligatures formed by the Miller's knot. The tails of the suture are placed down in a V formation to aid in forming the bump between the two ligatures of the knot, prior to tying the second ligature (Fig. 9.9).
- Tie a Second Ligature
  The second ligature is tied leaving space between it and the first ligature, so that a bump is formed between the two. The knot is secured with three throws (Fig. 9.10).
- Add a Third Ligature
  Next, one end of the suture is wrapped around the pedicle one more time, and another knot is tied with three throws. This modified Miller's knot then forms three ligatures around the pedicle (Fig. 9.11).

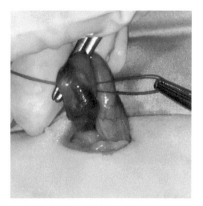

Fig. 9.7   Making a loop.

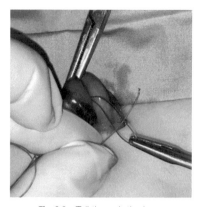

Fig. 9.8   Tail through the loop.

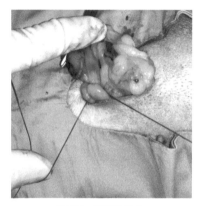

Fig. 9.9   First ligature.

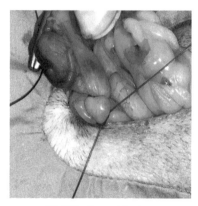

Fig. 9.10   Second ligature.

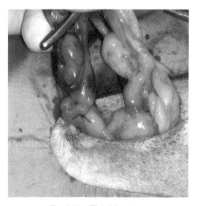

Fig. 9.11   Third ligature.

Transect The Pedicle Cranial to the Ovary

Because of adherent fat and connective tissue, the ovary is not always visible. However, its location can be determined by palpation. A minimum of a clear 1/4-inch (6 mm), preferably more, is left between the ovary and the ligature, so that the pedicle can be cleanly transected. Leaving even a small amount of ovarian tissue in the patient can lead to ovarian cysts, persistent estrus, and stump pyometra. The ovarian pedicle is transected, leaving a minimum of a 1/8-inch tag (preferably more) on the ovarian pedicle caudal to the ligature (Fig. 9.12).

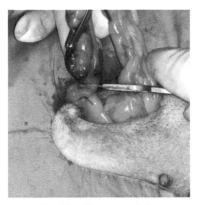

Fig. 9.12 Transect pedicle.

Detach The Mesometrium from The Uterus

The uterine artery is located lateral to the right horn. The surgeon's index finger is used to create a window in the mesometrium lateral to the artery. That window is extended laterally across the margin of the mesometrium portion of the broad ligament, and the mesometrium is detached from the uterus lateral to the uterine artery to the level of the uterine body.

Locate and Ligate The Left Ovary

The left horn is followed from the bifurcation to the left ovary. The previous steps are repeated for the left ovary.

Ligate The Two Uterine Arteries and The Uterus

The uterine arteries are ligated prior to ligating the uterus. Since a needle is required, the polydioxanone, that will later be used to close the abdomen, is used for this ligature.

- Place the suture around the arteries
  The needle is passed through the mesometrium, and under the artery, first on the far side of the uterus. Then it is passed over and through the uterus, under the artery on other side. See Figs 9.13 and 9.14 below.
- Tie the arterial ligature
  The ligature is tied with four throws, on the dorsal (upper) surface of the uterus. When tied, this places one ligature around both arteries See Fig 9.15 below.
- Ligate the Uterus
  A miller's knot is then placed around the uterus encompassing the arterial ligature. This results in the arteries, in effect, being triple ligated. See Fig 9.16 below.

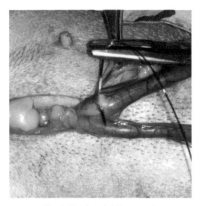

Fig. 9.13 Arterial ligature 1.

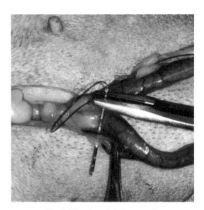

Fig. 9.14 Arterial ligature 2.

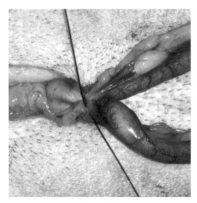

Fig. 9.15 Arterial ligature 3.

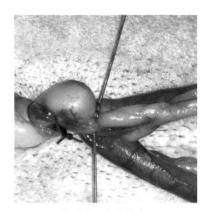

Fig. 9.16 Art/Miller's.

Transect The Uterus

Once the ligature is secure, transect the uterus cranial to the ligature and remove the ovaries and uterus, thus completing the ovariohysterectomy portion of the surgery.

Close The Linea Alba With A Continuous Cruciate Pattern

The linea is closed using a continuous cruciate pattern. The suture pattern starts and stops in the same place, making it possible to have just one knot. Because that one knot must therefore be extremely secure, two extra throws (for a total of six throws) are added to the knot and the suture ends are left long (a little less than 1/8 inch). For strength and durability, polydioxanone suture is used. Anticipating that the patient is likely to be more active postoperatively than is desirable, suture one size larger than is normally used in general practice is utilized (size 0 in large canines).

  ▪ First Bite

    A full-thickness bite is taken in the caudal end of the incision. The bite begins in the muscle adjacent to the linea on the far side from the surgeon and passes full thickness through the muscle. The needle is then passed across the incision, up through the muscle on the side of the incision nearest the surgeon (Fig. 9.17).

- Additional Bites

  A second identical bite is taken in the middle of the incision and another at the cranial end of the incision. If your incision is longer than 1.5 in (3.8 cm), continue the pattern until the cranial end of the incision is reached (Figs. 9.18 and 9.19).

  This forms two half cruciates (Fig. 9.20).

- Form the First Complete Cruciate

  The next bite crosses to the other side of the incision. The bite begins in the middle of the incision in the muscle adjacent to the linea on the far side from the surgeon and passes full thickness through the muscle. The needle is then passed across the incision, up through the muscle on the side of the incision nearest the surgeon (Fig. 9.21).

- Complete the Continuous Cruciate Pattern

  Another identical bite is taken at the caudal end of the incision. The two ends of the suture are tied together to form the second complete cruciate. If your incision is longer than 1.5 in (3.8 cm), form as many cruciate sutures as needed to close it (Fig. 9.22).

- Apply Six Throws

  Since this pattern does not have a knot at the beginning, it acts like a purse string if pulled tight. For that reason, the ends are not pulled tight until after the third throw. Six throws are applied for security (Fig. 9.23).

- Leave the Tags Long

  For extra security, the tags on the knot are left approximately 1/8 inch long (Fig. 9.24).

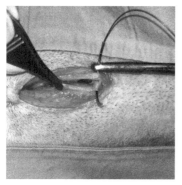

Fig. 9.17 Continuous cruciate first bite.

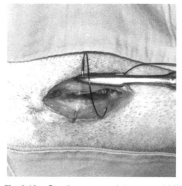

Fig. 9.18 Continuous cruciate second bite.

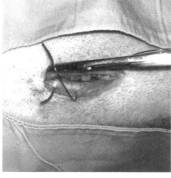

Fig. 9.19 Continuous cruciate third bite.

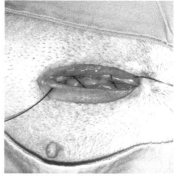

Fig. 9.20 Half cruciates.

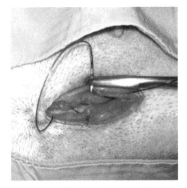

Fig. 9.21   First complete cruciate.

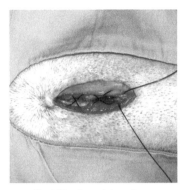

Fig. 9.22   Complete pattern.

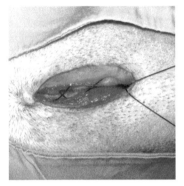

Fig. 9.23   Six throws.

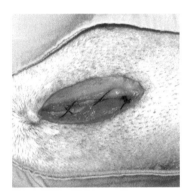

Fig. 9.24   Long tags.

Close The Subcuticular Tissue With a Continuous Subcuticular Pattern

The subcuticular tissue is closed with polydioxanone in a continuous subcuticular suture pattern with one knot. Since this pattern has only one knot, it will gather up like a purse string if it is tightened too soon. The suture is not pulled tight until after the third throw is placed. One extra throw is added to this knot, but the suture ends are cut off even with the knot. If any more throws are added or the ends are left long, the knot will not bury properly.

- First Bite
  The first bite starts deep, on the side nearest the surgeon, and comes up just under the skin at the cranial end of the incision (Fig. 9.25).
- Second Bite
  The needle is moved to the opposite side of the incision and a subcuticular bite is taken in a cranial to caudal direction (Fig. 9.26).
- Last Bites
  The needle is moved to the near side of the incision and a subcuticular bite is taken in a cranial to caudal direction. If the incision is longer than 1.5 in (3.8 cm), the pattern is continued until the caudal end of the incision is reached (Fig. 9.27).
  The last bite is taken in the opposite side of the incision from just under the skin and goes deep (Fig. 9.28).

■ The Knot

Since this suture has only one knot, it will gather up like a purse string if it is tightened too soon.

The suture is not pulled tight until after the third throw is placed. One extra throw is added to this knot (for a total of five throws). The suture ends are cut off even with the knot.

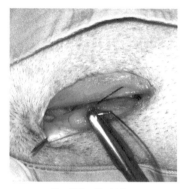

Fig. 9.25 First bite.

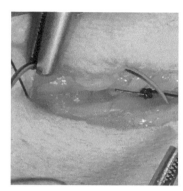

Fig. 9.26 Second bite.

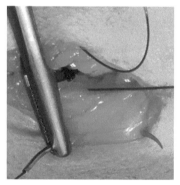

Fig. 9.27 Third bite.

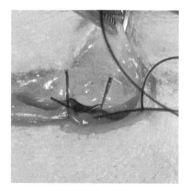

Fig. 9.28 Last bite.

Consider Applying A Tattoo

A small dot of green tattoo ink is applied to the cranial portion of the skin incision (the opposite end of the incision from where the knot is). Tattooing the patient helps to prevent an unnecessary abdominal exploratory in the future and the inherent risks associated with it.

Apply Tissue Glue To The Skin

Tissue glue is applied to the skin, being careful to cover the tattoo ink so that it will not get all over the owner's car, clothes, and furniture. Also, for extra safety, a drop of glue is placed on the subcuticular suture's knot to make it more secure.

OTHER CONSIDERATIONS

Pregnancy or Pyometra

- Use Large Canine Protocol
  The large canine protocol should be used for all patients who have enlarged vessels due to pregnancy, estrus, or pyometra.
- Enlarge the Incision
  The incision must be large enough to allow the surgeon to manually retrieve the gravid uterus. The uterine tissue is very friable in late term, so the incision must be large enough to gently extract the uterus. It should be larger than the crosswise diameter of the fetuses. It does not have to be the longitudinal length of the fetuses.
- Do Not Use the Spay Hook
  The spay hook is not used because of possible damage to the fragile uterus or enlarged blood vessels.
- Record Trimester and Number of Fetuses
  When the patient is pregnant, owners often want to know how far along the patient was and how many offspring were present. It is a good idea to include this information in the surgical notes.
- Assess Fetal Age
  Because of the extreme variation in size among canines, it is not possible to measure length of gestation based on fetal size. In general, in the first trimester, the amniotic sacs are round or ovoid and separated. They become more elongated and convergent in the second trimester. This is an inexact measurement because the number of fetuses will also determine the amount of separation between amniotic sacs. Skeletons are palpable in the third trimester.

Lactation

When milk is present in the mammary glands, care must be taken to avoid incising the mammary tissue. If the glands are incised, milk will leak into the incision. This may delay healing and could lead to infection or dehiscence.

TROUBLESHOOTING

Bleeding from The Abdominal Incision

It is always best to make the abdominal incision directly along the linea alba. Cutting the abdominal muscles can result in bleeding both intraoperatively and postoperatively. It also causes more postoperative pain for the patient. However, sometimes, the incision ends up to one side or the other of the linea. If this occurs, steps can be taken to prevent further harm from being done.

- Hold the Blade With the Sharp Edge Away From the Muscles
  When making the initial incision in the linea, the blade is held with the cutting edge up, so that if the linea alba is missed, only the muscle capsule is incised, and the underlying muscles are not severed.
- Use Blunt Dissection
  If the linea is missed, the blade is set aside, and a Kelly is used to separate the muscle fibers down to the peritoneum. Using blunt dissection rather than the blade on the muscles will result in less trauma and less bleeding.
- Incise the Peritoneum
  The peritoneum is then grasped with a pair of thumb forceps and elevated. It is incised with the blade, again, held cutting-edge-up, to avoid incising any internal organs.

CHAPTER 10

Standard Feline Spay

Victoria Valdez, DVM

This chapter presents the protocol I use for a standard ventral approach feline spay. Prior to learning the autoligation technique, this is the protocol I used. You will notice I do not use the "three-clamp" method for my ligatures. I find multiple clamps get in my way. I can see what I am doing much better using only one clamp, and doing so has proven to be is safe and time efficient. Chapter 11 outlines the protocol for a feline spay using the autoligation method.

Make The Abdominal Incisions

A ventral midline incision is made in the skin halfway between the umbilicus and the pubis. Goal incision size is 0.75 inch (1.9 cm). Blunt dissection is used to reach the linea alba. An incision, equal in size, is then made through the linea alba. For both incisions, the blade is held with the sharp surface pointing up, to avoid incising abdominal organs (Fig. 10.1).

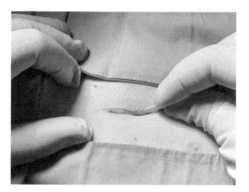

Fig. 10.1 Skin incision.

Exteriorize The Right Uterine Horn and Right Ovary

The right uterine horn is retrieved by sweeping the spay hook down the right abdominal wall to the dorsum directly perpendicular to the incision. The spay hook is then pulled medially, toward the incision, to engage the uterine horn. If what is engaged feels abnormally tight, it is possible the ureter is engaged. Release it and try again. It is common to hook the fat pad that lies lateral to the bladder. The uterine horn in the cat resides just cranial to that fat pad. If the fat pad is exteriorized, it is then held in place with a clamp and the spay hook is used to reach in just cranial to the fat pad and engage the uterine horn. Once the horn is exteriorized, it is followed manually it to the ovary (Fig. 10.2).

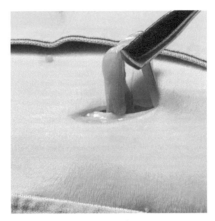

Fig. 10.2 Exteriorize ovary.

Ready The Right Ovarian Pedicle for Ligation

The surgeon's index finger is used to make a window in the mesovarium adjacent to the proper ligament. It is not necessary to extend the window cranially along the ovarian pedicle; it will automatically stretch to do this. This window is necessary for a ligature to be placed around the ovarian pedicle (Fig. 10.3).

A clamp is placed on the proper ligament of the right ovary (Fig. 10.4).

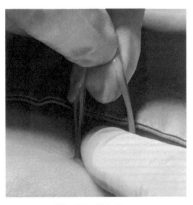

Fig. 10.3 Window.

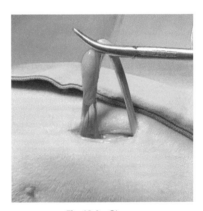

Fig. 10.4 Clamp.

Loosen or Break The Suspensory Ligament

If loosening the suspensory ligament is necessary to adequately exteriorize the ovary, gentle longitudinal digital pressure is exerted along the suspensory ligament to achieve this.

Ligate The Ovarian Pedicle with a Miller's Knot

Once the ovary is exposed well enough for good visualization, the right ovarian pedicle is ligated using a Miller's knot (see Fig. 9.2). A minimum of a clear 1/4 inch (6 mm), preferably more, is left between the ovary and the ligature, so that the pedicle can be cleanly transected. Leaving even a small amount of ovarian tissue in the patient can lead to ovarian cysts, persistent estrus, and stump pyometra. Chromic gut is used for security. Because it has relatively little memory, it is less likely than newer suture materials to come untied. Another advantage of chromic gut is that it requires only three throws on each knot. Because the surgeon needs to be able to really tighten the knots without the suture breaking, larger than normal gauge suture is used. 2-0 chromic gut works well in cats.

- Make a Loop in the Suture
  Using an approximate 16–18 inches of suture, a 4-inch loop is made in one end of the suture. The loop is placed on the far side of the pedicle (Fig. 10.5).
- Place One Tail Through the Loop
  One tail of the suture is placed through the loop and grasped with needle holders (Fig. 10.6).
- Place the First Ligature
  The suture is slid to the desired location below the ovary. Because of adherent fat and connective tissue, the ovary is not always visible. However, its location can be determined by palpation. A minimum of a clear 1/4 inch (6 mm), preferably more, is left between the ovary and the ligature, so that the pedicle can be cleanly transected. Leaving even a small amount of ovarian tissue in the patient can lead to ovarian cysts, persistent estrus, and stump pyometra. Pulling the two tails of the suture in opposite directions secures the first of the two ligatures formed by one Miller's knot (Fig. 10.7).
- Adjust the Suture
  The tails of the suture are placed up in a V formation to aid in forming the bump between the two ligatures (Fig. 10.8).
- Tie the Second Ligature
  The second ligature is tied, leaving space between it and the first ligature, so that a bump is formed between the two (Fig. 10.9).
- Complete the Knot
  The knot is completed with three throws and the sutures are clipped (Fig. 10.10).

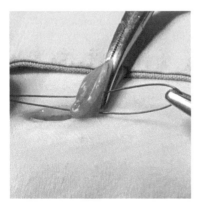

Fig. 10.5　Making a loop.

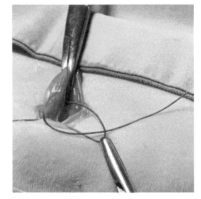

Fig. 10.6　Tail through the loop.

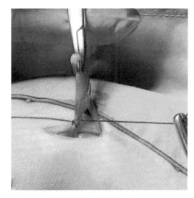

Fig. 10.7 First ligature.

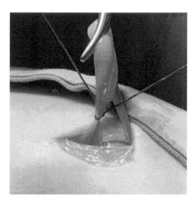

Fig. 10.8 Form a V.

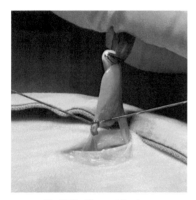

Fig. 10.9 Second ligature.

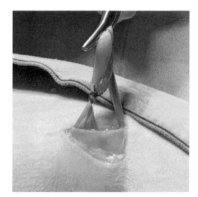

Fig. 10.10 Complete the knot.

Transect The Ovarian Pedicle

The ovarian pedicle is transected cranial to the ovary, leaving a minimum of a 1/8-inch tag (or more) on the pedicle caudal to the ligature (Fig. 10.11).

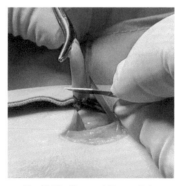

Fig. 10.11 Transect the pedicle.

Detach The Mesometrium from The Uterus

The uterine artery is located lateral to the right horn (Fig. 10.12).

The surgeon's index finger is used to create a window in the mesometrium lateral to the artery (Fig. 10.13).

The window in Fig. 10.13 is extended laterally across the margin of the mesometrium portion of the broad ligament, and the mesometrium is detached from the uterus lateral to the uterine artery to the level of the uterine body (Fig. 10.14).

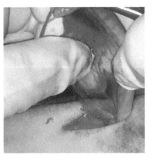

Fig. 10.12 Locate the artery.

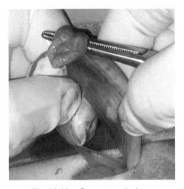

Fig. 10.13 Create a window.

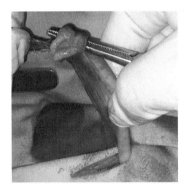

Fig. 10.14 Detach the mesometrium.

Locate and Ligate The Left Ovary

The left horn is followed from the bifurcation to the left ovary. The previous steps are repeated for the left ovary.

Ligate The Uterus with a Miller's Knot

The uterus is ligated using a Miller's knot of 2-0 chromic gut, cranial to the cervix. Another advantage of using a larger-diameter suture in the cat is that it is less likely to cut through the turgid uterus of the cat that is in estrus (Fig. 10.15).

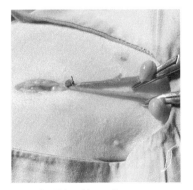

Fig. 10.15 Ligate the uterus.

Transect The Uterus

Once the ligature is secure, transect the uterus cranial to the ligature and remove the ovaries and uterus, thus completing the ovariohysterectomy portion of the surgery.

Close The Linea Alba With a Cruciate Suture

The linea is closed using a cruciate suture. Note: If your incision is longer than 0.75 inches, refer to Chapter 9, Large Canine Spay, for instructions on how to do a continuous cruciate pattern. The cruciate suture starts and stops in the same place, making it possible to have just one knot. Because that one knot must therefore be extremely secure, two extra throws are added to the knot (for a total of six throws) and the suture ends are left long (a little less than one-eighth inch). For strength and durability, polydioxanone suture is used. Anticipating that the patient is likely to be more active postoperatively than is desirable, suture one size larger than is normally used in general practice is utilized. For all cats, 2-0 polydioxanone is used.

- First Bite
  A full-thickness bite is taken in the caudal end of the incision. The bite begins in muscle adjacent to the linea on the far side from the surgeon. The needle is then passed across the incision, up through the muscle adjacent to the other side of the linea (Fig. 10.16).
- Second Bite
  A second identical bite is taken at the cranial end of the incision (Fig. 10.17).
  This forms a half cruciate (Fig. 10.18).
- Form Complete Cruciate
  The two ends of the suture are tied together to form the complete cruciate (Fig. 10.19).
- Apply Six Throws
  Since this pattern does not have a knot at the beginning, it acts like a purse string if pulled tight. For that reason, the ends are not pulled tight until after the third throw. Six throws are applied for security (Fig. 10.20).
- Leave the Tags Long
  For extra security, the tags on the knot are left approximately 1/8-inch long (Fig. 10.21).

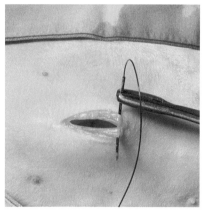

Fig. 10.16 Cruciate first bite.

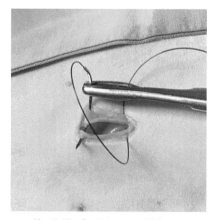

Fig. 10.17 Cruciate second bite.

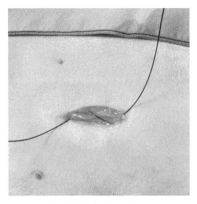

Fig. 10.18 Half cruciate.

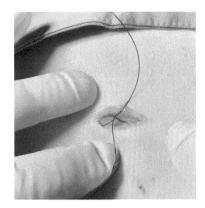

Fig. 10.19 Complete cruciate.

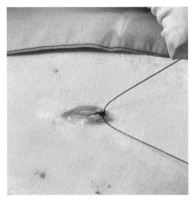

Fig. 10.20 Six throws.

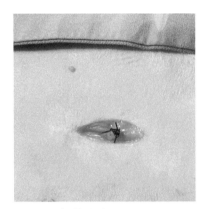

Fig. 10.21 Long tags.

Close The Skin With A Subcuticular Mattress Suture

The skin is closed with polydioxanone with a subcuticular mattress suture with one knot.

■ First Bite
   The first bite starts deep at the caudal end of the incision, on the side nearest the surgeon, and comes up just under the skin at the cranial end of the incision (Fig. 10.22).

■ Second Bite
   The needle is moved to the opposite side of the incision and a subcuticular bite is taken in a cranial to caudal direction (Fig. 10.23).

■ The Knot
   Since this suture has only one knot, it will gather up like a purse string if it is tightened too soon.
   The suture is not pulled tight until after the third throw is placed. One extra throw is added to this knot (for a total of five throws) (Fig. 10.24).

■ The Suture Ends
   The suture ends are cut off even with the knot. If any more throws are added or the ends are left long, the knot will not bury properly (Fig. 10.25).

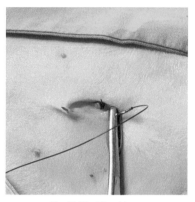

Fig. 10.22 First bite.

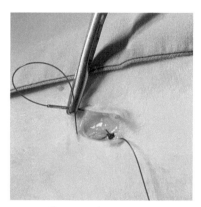

Fig. 10.23 Second bite.

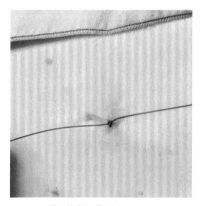

Fig. 10.24 Five throws.

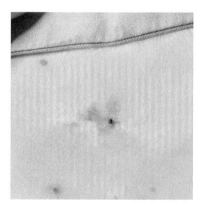

Fig. 10.25 Ends short.

Consider Applying A Tattoo

A small dot of green tattoo ink is applied to the cranial portion of the skin incision (the opposite end of the incision from where the knot is). Tattooing the patient helps to prevent an unnecessary abdominal exploratory in the future and the inherent risks associated with it.

Apply Tissue Glue To The Skin

Tissue glue is applied to the skin, being careful to cover the tattoo ink so that it will not stain the owner's car, clothes, and furniture. Also, for extra safety, a drop of glue is placed on the subcuticular suture's knot to make it more secure.

OTHER CONSIDERATIONS

Maintaining Statistics

When applying for grants for nonprofit spay/neuter programs, the following statistics are often helpful: how many cats were neutered, how many of those were in estrus, and how many were pregnant and with how many fetuses. The reproductive status of the female cat, and how many embryos or fetuses were present, as well as their gestational age should be included in the surgical notes (preferably in a manner in which they can be easily tabulated and retrieved for statistical purposes.)

Determining Gestational Age of Feline Fetuses in Utero (Table 10.1)

TABLE 10.1 ■ Quick Guide to Feline Gestational Age

Age in Weeks	Description, as Relates to Amniotic Sacs	Shape	Size
1	Not visible	N/A	N/A
2	Bumps in the road	Flat	0.25 in, 6 mm
3	Small green grapes	Ovoid	0.75 in, 18 mm
4	Larger purple grapes	Ovoid	1 in, 25 mm
5	Ping-pong ball to golf ball sized	Round	1.5 in, 40 mm–1.7 in, 43 mm
6	Become elongated/small gherkin sized Fetus is palpable	Elongated	2.5 in, 6 cm
7	As above but larger. Sacs converge Skull hardened	Elongated	3 in, 7.5 cm
8	As above but larger	Elongated	3.5 in, 9 cm
9	As above but larger (weigh 3.5–4 oz, 100–115 g at birth)	Elongated	4 in, 10.2 cm

Determining Estrus Status in a Feline

- No Sanguinous Discharge
  Since cats do not often show a sanguinous vaginal discharge while in heat, other factors must be evaluated.
- Behavioral Signs
  The owner may or may not recognize that a cat is in estrus based on behavioral signs such as vocalization and posturing.
- Appearance of the Uterus
  A more reliable method of determining estrus in a cat is examination of the uterus and ovaries during surgery. If the cat is in estrus, the uterus, when first exteriorized, will be white and glistening. (After it is handled a while, it will become red like a nonestrus uterus.) It will also be turgid, and therefore it is possible to cut through the tissue if ligatures are pulled too tight.
- Appearance of the ovaries
  The ovaries will contain multiple 2–4-mm fluid-filled, mature follicles or corpus luteum. Fig. 10.26 shows the turgid glistening uterus with a whitish appearance. The ovary contains multiple mature follicles.

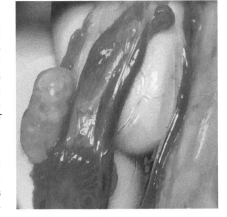

Fig. 10.26 Cat in estrus.

TROUBLESHOOTING

Postpartum Patients

The uterus is very friable in postpartum females. Care must be taken to not tug even slightly on the uterine horns or they may break. Since these cats often have milk in their mammary glands, care must also be taken to not incise these glands (see below).

Lactation

When milk is present in the mammary glands, care must be taken to avoid incising the mammary tissue. If the glands are incised, milk will leak into the incision. This will delay healing and could lead to infection or dehiscence.

- Manually Separate the Glands
  Prior to the midline skin incision, the surgeon runs his or her index finger down the midline between the two mammary chains to manually separate them.
- Make the Midline Incisions
  With the blade held with the sharp edge up, a stab wound is made just through the skin. The incision is carefully enlarged by incising the skin only and avoiding the underlying mammary tissue. The glands are separated by careful blunt dissection down to the linea alba. The linea is carefully incised, and the surgery continues as described earlier.
- Close the Midline Incisions
  When closing the linea alba, care is taken to avoid incising or puncturing the mammary tissue with a needle. A subcuticular mattress suture is used (as described) to close the skin. A subcuticular pattern involves placing sutures in the subcuticular tissue and avoids underlying tissues, in this case the mammary glands.

Cannot Expose The Uterine Bifurcation

- Check for Retained Mesometrium
  The lateral sides of the uterine horns are checked for retained mesometrium, and if present, it is removed. Even a small amount can tighten the horns and keep them from stretching, making it difficult to exteriorize the bifurcation.
- Use the Spay Hook as a Retractor
  The spay hook is placed in the incision in the linea alba and the abdominal wall is pulled caudally to expose the bifurcation, so that it can be traced to the other ovary (Fig. 10.27).
- Extend the Incision
  If the above two steps are not successful, the incision is extended caudally until the bifurcation is exposed.

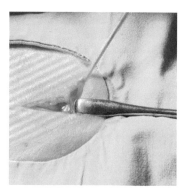

Fig. 10.27 Spay hook retractor.

CHAPTER 11

Auto-ligation Feline Spay

Victoria Valdez, DVM

An auto-ligation feline spay requires a very light hand, but with practice, it becomes second nature. The smaller the patient, the harder it is to do this surgery. For that reason, I recommend doing adult cats only until you feel comfortable with the procedure, then move on to kittens. I also used the "extra" clamp method, described below, for a full year before I felt secure enough to forgo the "extra" clamp. (It probably will not take you that long; I just tend to be overly cautious.) Putting into words the directions on how to do an auto-ligation spay makes it seem much more complicated than it really is. Once you have done it a few times, it will become one fluid motion. It cuts 2 minutes per surgery off the time required for a feline spay. That may not seem like much, but if you are doing 60 feline spays a day, that cuts 2 hours off your surgery time. It is well worth the effort to learn this safe, time-saving technique. The protocol I use is as follows.

PROTOCOL

Make The Abdominal Incisions

A ventral midline incision is made in the skin half way between the umbilicus and the pubis. Goal incision size is 0.75 inch (1.9 cm) (Fig. 11.1).

Blunt dissection is used to reach the linea alba. An incision, equal in size, is then made through the linea alba. For both incisions, the blade is held with the sharp surface pointing up, to avoid incising abdominal organs (Fig. 11.2).

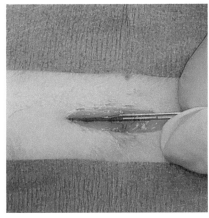

Fig. 11.1 Skin incision.

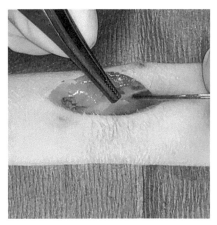

Fig. 11.2 Linea incision.

Exteriorize The Right Uterine Horn

The right uterine horn is retrieved by sweeping the spay hook down the right abdominal wall to the dorsum directly perpendicular to the incision (Fig. 11. 3).

The spay hook is then pulled medially, toward the incision, to engage the uterine horn. If what is engaged feels abnormally tight, it is possible the ureter is engaged. Release it and try again. It is common to hook the fat pad that lies lateral to the bladder. The uterine horn in the cat resides just cranial to that fat pad. If the fat pad is exteriorized, it is then held in place with a clamp and the spay hook is used to reach in just cranial to the fat pad and engage the uterine horn. Once the horn is exteriorized, it is followed manually to the ovary (Fig. 11.4).

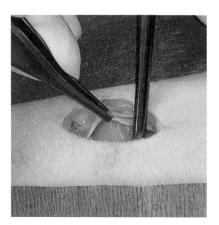 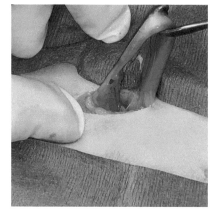

Fig. 11.3   Exteriorize horn.   **Fig. 11.4**   Spay hook.

Perform an Auto-Ligation

- Fan Out The Ovarian Pedicle
  Once the ovary is exteriorized, it is grasped with the surgeon's nondominant hand. The dominant hand is used to fan out the mesovarium such that the suspensory ligament is on the surgeon's left and the uterine horn is on the surgeon's right (Fig. 11.5).
- Cut The Suspensory Ligament
  The suspensory ligament is cut cranial to the ovary. The surgeon's index finger or the needle holders are used to make a window in the mesovarium between the ovarian vessels and the uterine artery (Fig. 11.6).
- Position The Uterine Horn
  With his or her nondominant hand, the surgeon very gently grasps the uterine horn about a 1/2 to 3/4 inch above the ovary and lays it down as it is pulled it toward him or her (Fig. 11.7).
- Position The Needle Holders
  The surgeon pictures a clock face lying on top of the pedicle with the pedicle stretching from 12 o'clock to 6 o'clock (the ovary being at 6 o'clock). With the surgeon's dominant hand, the needle holders (needle holders are used instead of a smaller clamp so that the knot the surgeon is going to make will slide off more easily.) are laid on top of the ovarian pedicle pointing roughly from 4 o'clock to 10 o'clock (Fig. 11.8).
- Wrap The Pedicle Around The Needle Holders
  The point of the needle holders is inserted *under* the pedicle from the left side, so that the needle holders point to 12 o'clock (Fig. 11.9).

- Rotate The Needle Holders

  Then, keeping the needle holders in the same plain as the imaginary clock, the point of the needle holders is rotated *over* the pedicle, counterclockwise, 180 degrees, so that it is pointing to 6 o'clock (Fig. 11.10).

- Grasp The Pedicle

  Next, the pedicle is grasped with the needle holders cranial to the ovary, leaving at least one quarter of an inch between the needle holders and the ovary. The needle holders are placed in the fully locked position (Fig. 11.11).

- Clamp The Proper Ligament

  A clamp is placed on the proper ligament of the ovary for hemostasis (Fig. 11.12).

- Use The Extra Clamp Method if Needed

  If the surgeon is new to using the auto-ligation technique, it is best at this point that a mosquito forceps is placed on the ovarian pedicle on the other side of the needle holders from the ovary. The mosquito is placed in the fully locked position. The more experienced surgeon skips this step and moves on to the next step (Fig. 11.13).

- Transect The Ovarian Pedicle

  The ovarian pedicle is transected between the ovary and the knot (Fig. 11.14).

- Slide The Knot Off The Needle Holders

  The knot is slid over and off the needle holders. It may help to use a piece of gauze over the knot for traction (Fig. 11.15).

- Secure The Knot

  Rather than tugging on the knot at this point to tighten it, it is pinched between the surgeon's thumb and index finger to flatten it, and while it is pinched, it is gently tugged to tighten it (Fig. 11.16).

- Remove The Extra Clamp

  Once it is determined that the knot is secure, the extra clamp is removed and the pedicle is allowed to slip back into the abdomen (Fig. 11.17).

- Revert To The Standard Method If Needed

  If, at any time during this method, the surgeon thinks that the pedicle feels like it might break, or the knot feels like it is slipping, he or she can, and should, revert to the standard protocol, i.e., standard suture ligatures.

- Locate And Auto-Ligate The Left Ovary

  Manipulation of the mesometrium during auto-ligation is often enough to detach it from the uterine horn, but if any remains lateral to the ovarian artery, it is removed now. The left horn is followed from the bifurcation to the left ovary. The above auto-ligation steps are repeated for the left ovary.

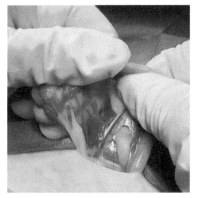
Fig. 11.5 Fan out pedicle.

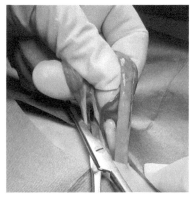
Fig. 11.6 Cut suspensory ligament.

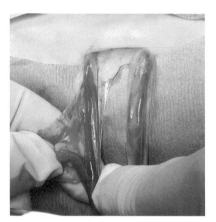

Fig. 11.7 Position the horn.

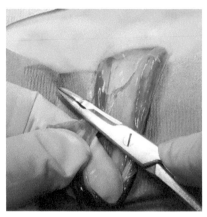

Fig. 11.8 Position the needle holders.

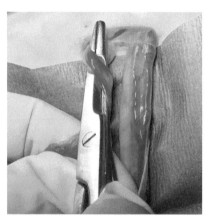

Fig. 11.9 Under the pedicle.

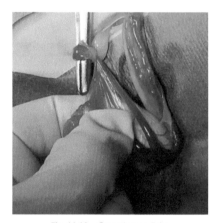

Fig. 11.10 Over the pedicle.

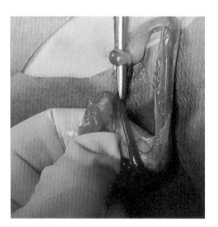

Fig. 11.11 Grasp the pedicle.

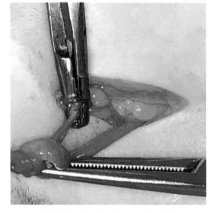

Fig. 11.12 Clamp proper ligament.

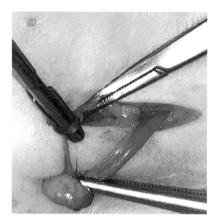

Fig. 11.13 Place extra clamp.

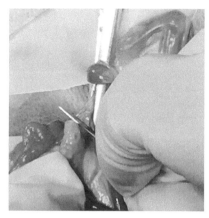

Fig. 11.14 Transect the pedicle.

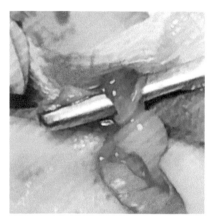

Fig. 11.15 Slide the knot.

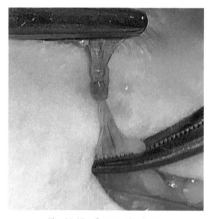

Fig. 11.16 Secure the knot.

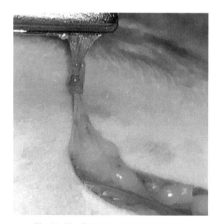

Fig. 11.17 Remove the extra clamp.

Ligate The Uterus With A Miller's Knot

The uterus is ligated using a Miller's knot of 2-0 chromic gut, cranial to the cervix. Another advantage of using larger diameter suture in the cat is that it is less likely to cut through the turgid uterus of the cat that is in estrus.

- Make a Loop in the Suture
  Using an approximate 16–18 inch of suture, a 4-inch loop is made in one end of the suture. The loop is placed on the far side of the pedicle (Fig. 11.18).
- Place One Tail Through the Loop
  One tail of the suture is placed through the loop and grasped with needle holders (Fig. 11.19).
- Place the First Ligature
  The suture is slid to the desired location below the ovary. Because of adherent fat and connective tissue, the ovary is not always visible. However, its location can be determined by palpation. A minimum of a clear 1/4 inch (6 mm), preferably more, is left between the ovary and the ligature, so that the pedicle can be cleanly transected. Leaving even a small amount of ovarian tissue in the patient can lead to ovarian cysts, persistent estrus, and stump pyometra. Pulling the two tails of the suture in opposite directions secures the first of the two ligatures formed by one Miller's knot (Fig. 11.20).
- Adjust the Ties
  The tails of the suture are placed up in a V formation to aid in forming the bump between the two ligatures (Fig. 11.21).
- Tie the Second Ligature
  The second ligature is tied, leaving space between it and the first ligature, so that a bump is formed between the two (Fig. 11.22).
- Complete the knot and transect the uterus
  The knot is completed with three throws, the sutures are clipped and the uterus is transected (Fig. 11.23).

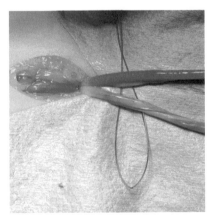

Fig. 11.18 Making a loop.

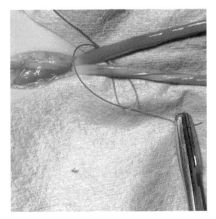

Fig. 11.19 Tail through the loop.

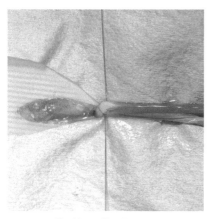

Fig. 11.20   First ligature.

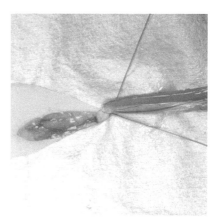

Fig. 11.21   Adjust the ties.

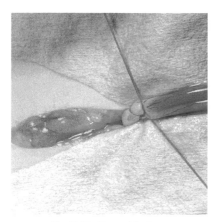

Fig. 11.22   Second ligature.

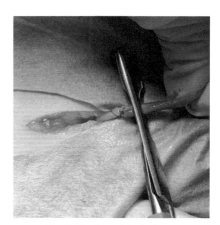

Fig. 11.23   Complete the knot.

Close The Linea Alba With A Cruciate Suture

The linea is closed using a cruciate suture. Note: If your incision is longer than 0.75 inch, refer to Chapter 9, Large Canine Spay, for instructions on how to do a continuous cruciate pattern. The cruciate suture starts and stops in the same place, making it possible to have just one knot. Because that one knot must therefore be extremely secure, two extra throws are added to the knot (for a total of six throws) and the suture ends are left long (a little less than 1/8 inch). For strength and durability, polydioxanone suture is used. Anticipating that the patient is likely to be more active postop than is desirable, suture one size larger than is normally used in general practice is utilized. For all cats, 2-0 polydioxanone is used.

- First Bite

  A full-thickness bite is taken in the caudal end of the incision. The bite begins in the linea on the far side from the surgeon and passes full thickness through the linea. The needle is then is passed across the incision, up through the linea on the side of the incision nearest the surgeon (Fig. 11.24).

- Second Bite
  A second identical bite is taken at the cranial end of the incision (Fig. 11.25).
  This forms a half cruciate (Fig. 11.26).
- Form Complete Cruciate
  The two ends of the suture are tied together to form the complete cruciate (Fig. 11.27).
- Apply Six Throws
  Since this pattern does not have a knot at the beginning, it acts like a purse string if pulled
  tight. For that reason, the ends are not pulled tight until after the third throw. Six throws
  are applied for security (Fig. 11.28).
- Leave the Tags Long
  For extra security, the tags on the knot are left approximately 1/8 inch long (Fig. 11.29).

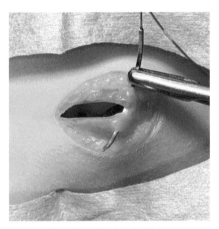

Fig. 11.24 Cruciate first bite.

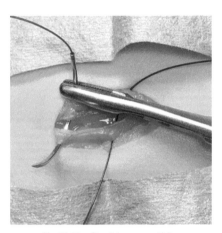

Fig. 11.25 Cruciate second bite.

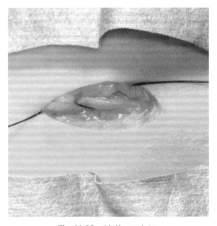

Fig. 11.26 Half cruciate.

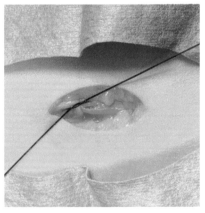

Fig. 11.27 Complete cruciate.

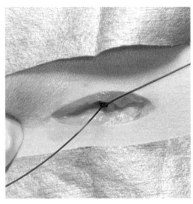

Fig. 11.28 Six throws.

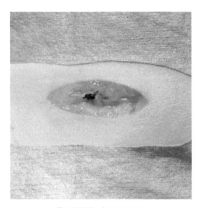

Fig. 11.29 Long tags.

Close The Skin With A Subcuticular Mattress Suture

The skin is closed with polydioxanone with a subcuticular mattress suture with one knot.

- First Bite

  The first bite starts deep at the caudal end of the incision, on the side nearest the surgeon, and comes up just under the skin at the cranial end of the incision (Fig. 11.30).
- Second Bite

  The needle is moved to the opposite side of the incision and a subcuticular bite is taken in a cranial to caudal direction (Fig. 11.31).
- The Knot

  Since this suture has only one knot, it will gather up like a purse string if it is tightened too soon. The suture is not pulled tight until after the third throw is placed. One extra throw is added to this knot (for a total of five throws) (Fig. 11.32).
- The Suture Ends

  The suture ends are cut off even with the knot. If any more throws are added or the ends are left long, the knot will not bury properly (Fig. 11.33).

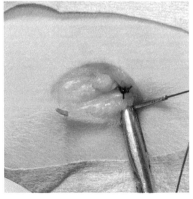

Fig. 11.30 First bite.

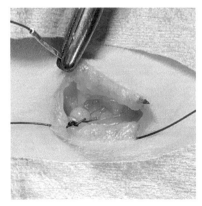

Fig. 11.31 Second bite.

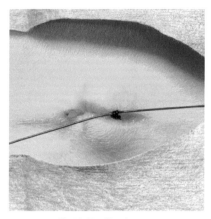

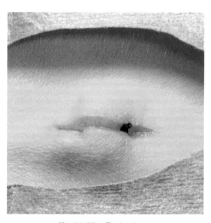

Fig. 11.32 Five throws.   **Fig. 11.33** Ends short.

Consider Applying A Tattoo

A small dot of green tattoo ink is applied to the cranial portion of the skin incision (the opposite end of the incision from where the knot is). Tattooing the patient helps to prevent an unnecessary abdominal exploratory in the future and the inherent risks associated with it.

Apply Tissue Glue To The Skin

Tissue glue is applied to the skin being careful to cover the tattoo ink so that it will not stain the owner's car, clothes, and furniture. Also, for extra safety, a drop of glue is placed on the subcuticular suture's knot to make it more secure. Once the glue is applied, the skin edges are apposed and held in place a few seconds to bury the knot (Fig. 11.34).

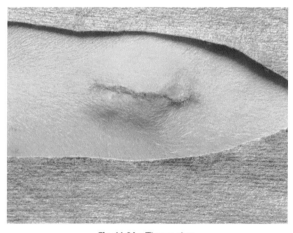

Fig. 11.34 Tissue glue.

OTHER CONSIDERATIONS

Maintaining Statistics

When applying for grants for nonprofit spay/neuter programs, the following statistics are often helpful: how many cats were neutered, how many of those were in estrus, and how many were pregnant and with how many fetuses. The reproductive status of the female cat, and how many embryos or fetuses were present, as well as their gestational age, should be included in the surgical notes (preferably, in a manner in which they can be easily tabulated and retrieved for statistical purposes.)

Determining Gestational Age of Feline Fetuses in Utero (Table 11.1)

TABLE 11.1 ■ Quick Guide to Feline Gestational Age

Age in Weeks	Description, as Relates to Amniotic Sacs	Shape	Size
1	Not visible	N/A	N/A
2	Bumps in the road	Flat	0.25 in, 6 mm
3	Small green grapes	Ovoid	0.75 in, 18 mm
4	Larger purple grapes	Ovoid	1 in, 25 mm
5	Ping-pong ball to golf ball sized	Round	1.5 in, 40 mm–1.7 in, 43 mm
6	Become elongated/small gherkin sized Fetus is palpable	Elongated	2.5 in, 6 cm
7	As above but larger. Sacs converge Skull hardened	Elongated	3 in, 7.5 cm
8	As above but larger	Elongated	3.5 in, 9 cm
9	As above but larger (weigh 3.5–4 oz, 100–115 g at birth)	Elongated	4 in, 10.2 cm

Determining Estrus Status In A Feline

- No Sanguinous Discharge
  Since cats do not often show a sanguinous vaginal discharge while in heat, other factors must be evaluated.
- Behavioral Signs
  The owner may or may not recognize that a cat is in estrus based on behavioral signs such as vocalization and posturing.
- Appearance of the Uterus
  A more reliable method of determining estrus in a cat is examination of the uterus and ovaries during surgery. If the cat is in estrus, the uterus, when first exteriorized, will be white and glistening. (After it is handled a while, it will become red like a nonestrus uterus.) It will also be turgid, and therefore it is possible to cut through the tissue if ligatures are pulled too tight.
- Appearance of the Ovaries
  The ovaries will contain multiple 2–4-mm fluid-filled, mature follicles or corpus luteum.
  Fig. 11.35 shows the turgid glistening uterus with a whitish appearance. The ovary contains multiple mature follicles.

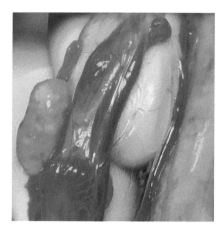

Fig. 11.35   Cat in estrus.

TROUBLESHOOTING

Delicate Ovarian Vessels in Very Small Kittens

In very small kittens, the ovarian vessels may be as thin as threads. (Note: I do not perform surgery on kittens less than 8 weeks old or on those that weigh less than 2 lb, or 0.9 kg.) The following modifications to the previous protocol may be necessary in these patients:

- Do Not Cut the Suspensory Ligament
  The suspensory ligament is not cut; instead it is incorporated into the knot of the auto-ligation.
- Use a Curved Mosquito Forceps
  A curved mosquito forceps is used to do the auto-ligation instead of the needle holders. It will be slightly more difficult to slide the knot off the instrument, but this is more than compensated for in the ease and safety of performing the auto-ligation on such delicate structures.

Abdominal Closure is not Flat

- Common in Felines
  This is a common problem in cats because of the extra fat they have under the skin in the ventral abdominal area.
- Remove the Fat at the Time the Initial Abdominal Incision Is Made
  Once the skin incision is made, if fat is present, it is grasped with forceps and removed with scissors from the area of the incision. The surgery then proceeds as given earlier.
- Flatten the Incision
  After closing the skin and applying a tattoo and tissue glue, a piece of gauze is placed over the incision, and it is quickly and gently tamped down manually to flatten the underlying fat.

CHAPTER 12

Canine Scrotal Neuter

Victoria Valdez, DVM

It is my clinical impression that the bigger the dog, the greater the chance of a scrotal hematoma.

I have found the most likely source of the bleeding to be from where the scrotal ligament was attached to the scrotum or from a small bleeder on the midline between the two peritesticular incisions. Given those two facts, I see no reason why a prescrotal surgery would be any safer than a scrotal one. In fact, the opposite should be true. However, I have learned that, in my hands, I see more complications with a scrotal technique than a prescrotal one. Therefore, I reserve a scrotal technique for puppies 10 lb or less who still have their deciduous canines. These dogs have a flatter-looking scrotum when they are in dorsal recumbency and testicles comparable in size to a cat or kitten (Fig. 12.1).

I ligate the spermatic cord with chromic gut rather than auto-ligate it because early in my career I had an auto-ligated cord come untied in a puppy and I never want to have that happen again. We are all products of our experience. I think that is why protocols vary so widely, and as surgeons, we all have our own personal preferences. If a scrotal approach works for you and you are not seeing any complications, then you should continue doing what you are doing. The protocol I use for a scrotal neuter is the following.

PROTOCOL

Make An Incision along The Scrotal Midline

The testicles are held in place on the midline of the scrotum. A skin incision is made through the ventral scrotum. The incision only has to be as long as the cross-sectional diameter of the testicle, i.e., long enough to extrude the testicle through it. Upward pressure is applied to the testicle as the scrotum is incised (Fig. 12.2).

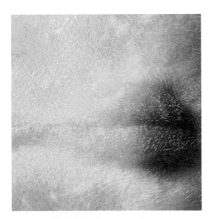

Fig. 12.1 Puppy scrotum.

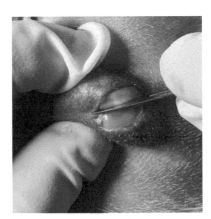

Fig. 12.2 Scrotal incision.

Exteriorize the Testicle

Gentle, even pressure is applied, and the testicle is pulled out of the incision, thereby exposing the spermatic cord. Too vigorous pulling of the spermatic cord can cause vessels deeper along the cord or on the lining of the scrotum to break and bleed. If the cord is not pulling easily, incise the fascia distal to the tail of the epididymis to loosen the ligamentous attachments to the parietal tunic.

Strip Fat from The Spermatic cord if Needed

If the cords are to be auto-ligated, fat is stripped from the cord. If the cords are to be ligated with suture, as they are in this protocol, manipulation of the cord is often enough to remove sufficient fat from it and stripping them is not necessary.

Exteriorize both testicles before applying ligatures

Both testicles are exteriorized prior to ligating and removing them so that it is impossible beyond this point to forget one testicle. If the surgeon is interrupted with an emergency at this point, he or she will know exactly where to resume the protocol when returning to surgery (Fig. 12.3).

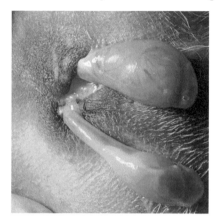

Fig. 12.3 Exteriorize both testicles.

Ligate the Spermatic Cords with Miller's Knots

Use a Miller's knot of 2-0 chromic gut to ligate each spermatic cord. This will in effect form two ligatures with a bump in between to keep the ligatures from sliding.

- Make a Loop in the Suture
  Using an approximate 16–18 inches of suture, a 4-inch loop is made in one end of the suture. The loop is placed on the far side of the spermatic cord (Fig. 12.4).
- Place One Tail Through the Loop
  One tail of the suture is placed through the loop and grasped with needle holders (Fig. 12.5).
- Tie the First Ligature
  The suture is slid to the desired location on the spermatic cord. Pulling the two tails of the suture in opposite directions secures the first of the two ligatures formed by one miller's knot. The tails of the suture are placed in an inverted-V formation to aid in forming the bump between the two ligatures of the knot, prior to tying the second ligature (Fig. 12.6).
- Tie the Second Ligature
  The second ligature is tied leaving space between it and the first ligature, so that a bump is formed between the two (Fig. 12.7).
- Secure With Three Throws
  The knot is completed with three throws and the sutures are clipped (Fig. 12.8).

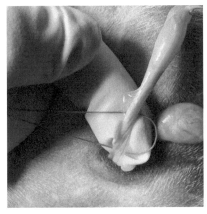

Fig. 12.4 Making a loop.

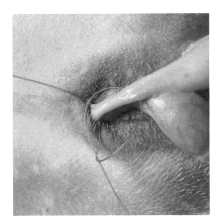

Fig. 12.5 Tail through the loop.

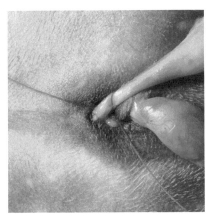

Fig. 12.6 First ligature.

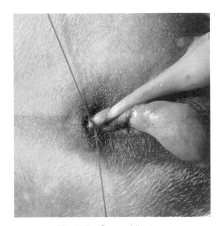

Fig. 12.7 Second ligature.

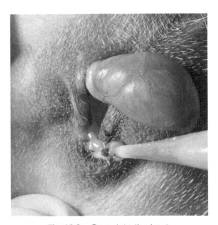

Fig. 12.8 Complete the knot.

Repeat for the other Spermatic cord and Transect the cords

When both spermatic cords are ligated, they are transected distal to the ligatures.

Close the Incision

The incision is checked to be sure no subcutaneous tissue or spermatic cord remnant is protruding into the incision. When the incision is clean, it is closed with tissue glue.

- Apply Glue to the Incision
  Tissue glue is applied to the skin being careful to cover the tattoo ink so that it won't stain the owner's car, clothes and furniture. Also, for extra safety, a drop of glue is placed on the subcuticular suture's knot to make it more secure (Fig. 12.9).
- Appose Skin Edges
  Appose the skin edges and hold in place a few seconds while the glue dries (Fig. 12.10).

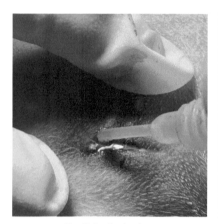 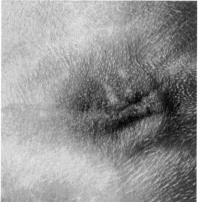

Fig. 12.9   Apply glue.   **Fig. 12.10**   Closure.

Consider a Tattoo

To prevent an unnecessary and invasive surgery in the future, consider applying a tattoo. Because the scrotum is often pigmented, the tattoo is placed in the prescrotal area to make the tattoo more visible.

- Make an Incision in the Prescrotal Area
  A separate short, shallow incision is made in the prescrotal area (Fig. 12.11).
- Apply Tattoo Ink
  It is not necessary to apply a long tattoo. Even a dot of green ink should alert the observer to the fact that the animal has been sterilized (Fig. 12.12).
- Apply Tissue Glue
  Tissue glue is applied over the ink to prevent it from staining the owner's clothes, car, and furniture (Fig. 12.13).
- Appose Edges
  Once the glue is applied, the skin edges are apposed and held in place a few seconds until the glue is dried (Fig. 12.14).

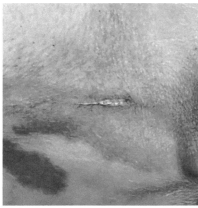

Fig. 12.11 Tattoo incision.

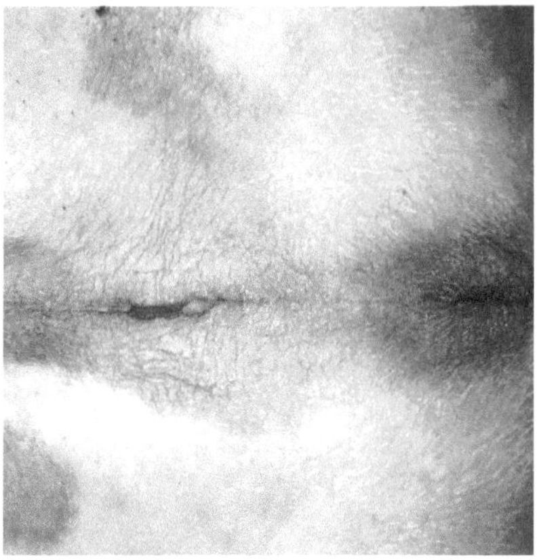

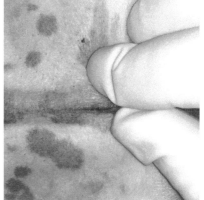

Fig. 12.12 Ink applied.

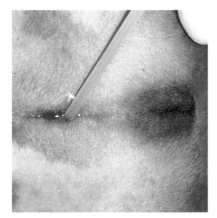

Fig. 12.13 Glue.

Fig. 12.14 Appose edges.

TROUBLESHOOTING

Abdominal fluid (ascites) is Present in the Scrotum

- Normal in Juveniles
  Ascites is "normal" in puppies (and kittens) due to the hypoproteinemia frequently present in young animals.
- Recommend Appropriate Diet
  Owners should be advised that if they are not already doing so, they need to feed a good-quality puppy (or kitten) food.

CHAPTER 13

Canine Prescrotal Neuter

Victoria Valdez, DVM

I use the prescrotal approach for all canine neuters (except puppies under 16 weeks and 10 lb or less). One of the most frequent complications seen in high-volume spay/neuter is a scrotal hematoma post neuter. A common causal factor related to this occurrence is hyperactivity. Those little vessels that are cut and clot during surgery can open back up and start bleeding when the patient is running or roughhousing after surgery. It is important to advise the owner to keep the patient quiet during the recovery period. Consider prescribing diphenhydramine during this period to achieve drowsiness (1 mg/lb orally bid x 5–7 days). Even if the patient is quiet, a scrotal hematoma can occur. It is important to incise as few vessels as possible and to achieve precise hemostasis and a secure closure.

I like to instill a drop of epinephrine in all my incisions to constrict the small vessels in the skin. It is especially helpful in a castration to differentiate small skin bleeders from those in deeper tissues. If bleeding is still occurring after application of epinephrine, I know it is from deeper vessels and I need to find and deal with those bleeders or they will cause trouble later.

Each surgeon has his or her own preferred canine neuter protocol. I use a prescrotal approach, closed technique.

CANINE PRESCROTAL NEUTER PROTOCOL

Position the First Testicle

One testicle is manually pushed craniad to the prescrotal area of the prepuce. The further cranially the incision is made, the thicker the overlying skin will be and the easier it will be to close (Figs. 13.1 and 13.2).

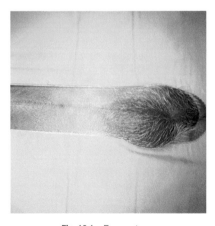

Fig. 13.1 Prescrotum.

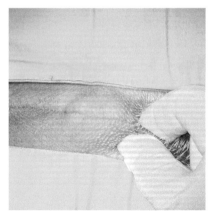

Fig. 13.2 Position testicle.

Make the Midline Incision

The testicle is held in place on the midline. An incision is made over the testicle, along the ventral midline. The incision only has to be as long as the cross-sectional diameter of the testicle; i.e., long enough to extrude the testicle through it. Making the incision directly over the midline without the testicle in place increases the risk of accidently incising the urethra, a rare but possible complication (Fig. 13.3).

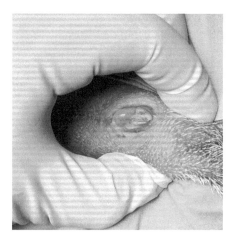

Fig. 13.3 Incision.

Incise Over the Testicles

Each testicle is held in turn, up into the midline incision, and the subcutaneous tissue and spermatic fascia are incised down to the level of the parietal vaginal tunic that covers it. Fat at this level usually serves as a helpful landmark, indicating the correct level has been reached. Any less deep, and the testicle cannot be exteriorized; any deeper, and the parenchyma of the testicle will be incised, causing bleeding and consequent loss of visibility of the surgery site (Fig. 13.4).

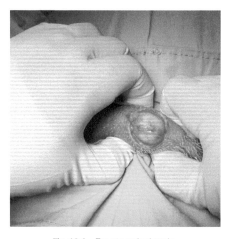

Fig. 13.4 Fat at vaginal tunic.

Exteriorize the Testicles

The length of each incision is extended as needed to extrude the testicle through it. An attempt is made to pull each testicle cranially, out through the incision with gentle, even traction. The ligament of the tail of the epididymis attaches the testicle to the tail of the epididymis and the scrotal ligament connects the testicle to the scrotum. In small or young animals these ligaments are often loose enough that it is possible to pull the testicles out of the incision without transecting the ligaments. Too vigorous pulling of the spermatic cord can cause vessels deeper along the cord or on the lining of the scrotum to break and bleed (Fig. 13.5).

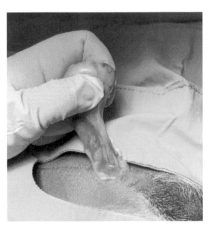

Fig. 13.5   Exteriorize testicle.

Transect the Ligaments If Needed

In older animals the ligaments are often tougher and will need to be severed. The testicle is elevated enough to visualize the tail of the epididymis. It is often possible to see through the fascia in this area to identify the ligament of the tail of the epididymis. Even if it is not readily visible, it is possible to incise it. The testicle is held with the surgeon's nondominant hand, with the epididymis on the far edge. A blade is used to fenestrate the fascia just below the testicle, in an area where it is translucent and contains no structures. The blade is then used to cut from the fenestration to the outer edge of the fascia, away from the spermatic cord (Fig. 13.6).

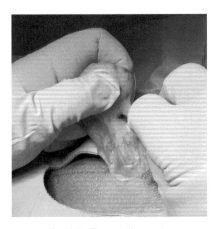

Fig. 13.6   Transect ligaments.

It is possible to feel the testicle free up as the ligaments are transected. Once the attachments are free, the spermatic cord is exposed by pulling the testicle cranially with gentle even pressure.

Remove Fat From the Spermatic Cord If Needed

Generally, manipulation of the cord is enough to remove sufficient fat from it, but in very large or obese animals, it might be necessary to remove excess fat from the spermatic cord before applying ligatures. Fat may be removed by drawing a clamp or a piece of gauze along the cord (Fig. 13.7).

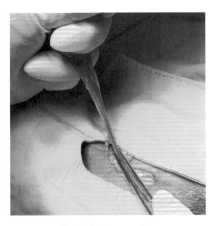

Fig. 13.7   Remove fat.

Exteriorize Both Testicles Before Applying Ligatures

Both testicles are exteriorized prior to ligating and removing them so that it is impossible beyond this point to forget one testicle. If the surgeon is interrupted with an emergency at this point, he or she will know exactly where to resume the protocol when returning to surgery (Fig. 13.8).

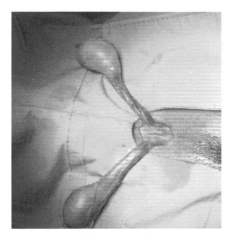

Fig. 13.8   Both testicles.

Ligate the Spermatic Cords Using Miller's Knots

Use a Miller's knot of 2-0 chromic gut to ligate each spermatic cord. Each knot will, in effect, form two ligatures with a bump in between to keep the ligatures from sliding.

- Make a Loop in the Suture

  Using an approximate 16–18 inches of suture, a 4-inch loop is made in one end of the suture. The loop is placed on the far side of the part requiring ligation (Fig. 13.9).

- Place One Tail Through the Loop

  One tail of the suture is placed through the loop and grasped with needle holders (Fig. 13.10).

- Tighten the First Ligature

  The suture is slid to the desired location on the spermatic cord. Pulling the two tails of the suture in opposite directions secures the first of the two ligatures formed by one Miller's knot (Fig. 13.11).

- Adjust Placement for Second Ligature

  The tails of the suture are placed in an inverted V formation to aid in forming the bump between the two ligatures of the knot, prior to tying the second ligature (Fig. 13.12).

- Tie Second Ligature

  The second ligature is tied leaving space between it and the first ligature, so that a bump is formed between the two (Fig. 13.13).

- Secure With Three Throws

  The knot is completed with three throws and the sutures are clipped (Fig. 13.14).

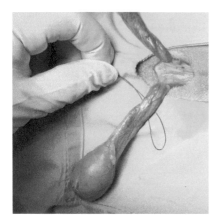

Fig. 13.9   Making a loop.

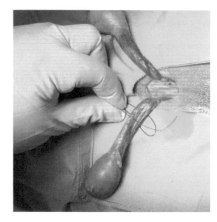

Fig. 13.10   Tail through the loop.

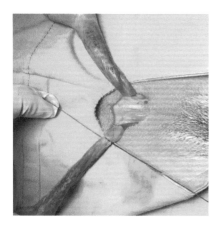

Fig. 13.11   First ligature.

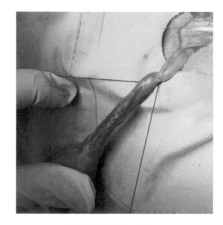

Fig. 13.12   Adjust ties.

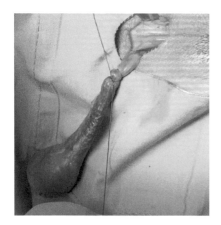

Fig. 13.13   Second ligature.

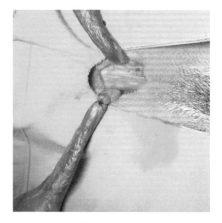

Fig. 13.14   Complete the knot.

Transect the Spermatic Cords

Each spermatic cord is transected leaving at least 1/8- to 1/4 inch tag of cord distal to the knot (Fig. 13.15).

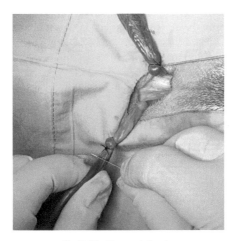

Fig 13.15 Transect Cords.

Close the Peri-Testicular Incisions

The peri-testicular incisions are closed with one continuous suture pattern of 2-0 polydioxanone with *no knot*.

- Start the closure by taking a bite in the far edge of the left peri-testicular incision, through the midline, to the far edge of the right peri-testicular incision (Fig. 13.16).
- Repeat this bite going cranially every 1/2 to 5/8 in. (1.25–1.5 cm) until the peri-testicular incisions are closed (Fig. 13.17).

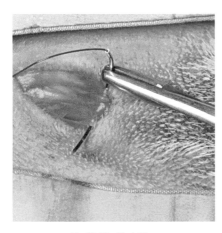

Fig 13.16 First Bite.

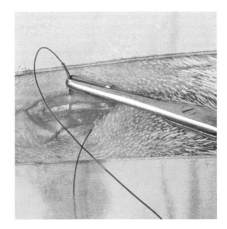

Fig 13.17 Additional Bites.

Close the Skin

Without placing a knot, the same suture is then used to close the skin in a subcuticular pattern.

- The first bite starts deep and comes up in the subcuticular tissue, just under the skin (Fig. 13.18).
- The next bite crosses to the other side of the incision and travels in the opposite direction. It starts and ends in the subcuticular tissue (Fig. 13.19).
- The last bite crosses back to the near side of the incision and starts in the subcuticular tissue but ends deep (Fig. 13.20).
- For security, an extra throw is added to the knot (for a total of five throws) (Fig. 13.21).

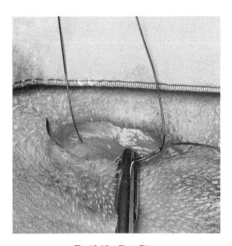

Fig 13.18   First Bite.

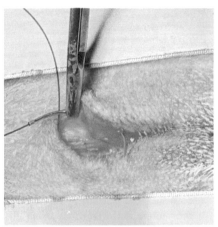

Fig 13.19   Second Bite.

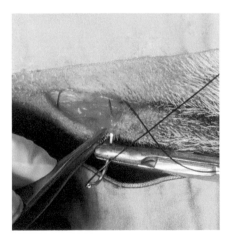

Fig. 13.20   Last bite.

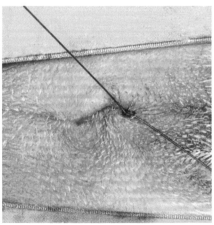

Fig. 13.21   Five Throws.

Consider Applying a Tattoo

A small dot of green tattoo ink is applied to the cranial portion of the skin incision (the opposite end of the incision from where the knot is). Tattooing the patient prevents an unnecessary abdominal exploratory in the future and the inherent risks associated with it.

Apply Tissue Glue to the Skin

Tissue glue is applied to the skin being careful to cover the tattoo ink so that it will not stain the owner's car, clothes, and furniture. Also, for extra safety, a drop of glue is placed on the subcuticular suture's knot to make it more secure.

TROUBLESHOOTING

Scrotal Bleeding

- Apply Epinephrine
  A drop of epinephrine in the incision site will cause small vessels in the skin to contract. This helps differentiate small skin bleeders from deeper vessels that may be bleeding.
- Common Sites of Bleeding
  The two most common sites of bleeding in a canine neuter done as described are from the site where the scrotal ligament attached to the scrotum and from the midline of the skin incision.
- Rule Out Bleeding From the Incision
  If any bleeders in the skin incision are found and either cauterized or ligated and bleeding is still occurring, it is most likely from the scrotum.
- Explore the Scrotum
  The blunt end of a blade holder or a spay hook is used to gently invert the scrotum and locate any bleeders. The bleeders are either cauterized or ligated for hemostasis.

Cannot Exteriorize the Testicle Enough to Sever Ligamentous Attachments

- Be Sure the Parietal Vaginal Tunic Is Exposed
  Fat is often, but not always, present at the level of the vaginal tunic. Incising any deeper than the vaginal tunic will puncture the testicular parenchyma, but this will prove that the parietal vaginal tunic has been reached.
- Individual Variation
  In some animals, especially older ones, the ligamentous attachments can be abnormally tough and tight.
- Incise the Tail of the Epididymis
  If it is not possible to elevate the testicle enough to visualize the area below the tail of the epididymis, the tail of the epididymis is incised until the surgeon can feel the testicle free up enough to cut the ligaments in the manner described above.

CHAPTER 14

Feline Neuter

Victoria Valdez, DVM

A feline neuter is a simple operation, and yet there are some subtle details that bear examining. It is not unusual for the scrotum to swell and bleed postoperatively in a cat. Paying close attention to each step of the surgery can alleviate this. With that in mind, the following protocol attempts to address those small details that can help prevent this post-operative complication.

PROTOCOL

Position the Patient

The patient is positioned in dorsal recumbency with the legs pulled up and back toward the head. One way to do this is as follows:

- A rubber band or cuff from a surgery glove is attached to one end of a surgery tie.
- The other end of the tie is attached to the head of the surgery table (Fig. 14.1).
- The rubber band or cuff is wrapped around the patient's back legs behind the hocks (Fig. 14.2).
- This elevates the testicles for easy access for surgery (Fig. 14.3).

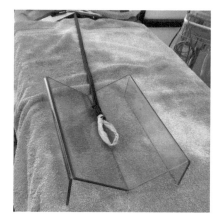

Fig. 14.1 Modified surgery tie.

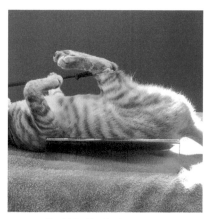

Fig. 14.2 Positioning the tie.

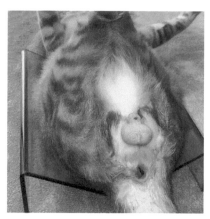

Fig. 14.3 Proper positioning of the testicles.

Anesthesia

Be sure the patient is fully anesthetized before making the scrotal incision. If the patient is light, his blood pressure is consequently higher. It is these patients that tend to bleed postoperatively.

Incise the Scrotum

One incision is made on the midline of the scrotum. One incision rather than two means less potential for bleeding (Figs. 14.4 and 14.5).

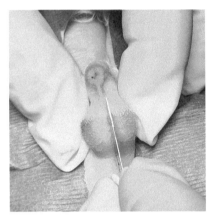

Fig. 14.4 Incise the scrotum.

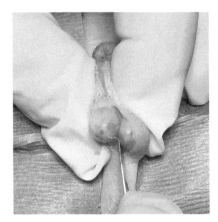

Fig. 14.5 Incise the scrotum.

Instill Epinephrine

A drop of epinephrine is used in the skin incision to constrict the small capillaries there (Fig. 14.6).

Incise over the Testicles

Incisions are then made over each testicle to free them from the overlying connective tissue (Fig. 14.7).

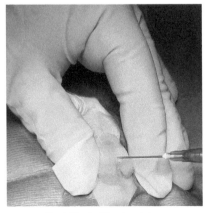

Fig. 14.6 Instill epinephrine.

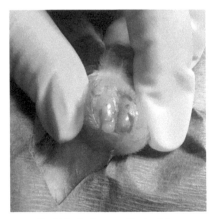

Fig. 14.7 Incise over the testicles.

Exteriorize the Testicle

Gentle, even traction is used to extrude the testicle and expose the spermatic cord. Too vigorous handling of the cords can cause them to break or cause breaking of vessels further up the cord (Fig. 14.8).

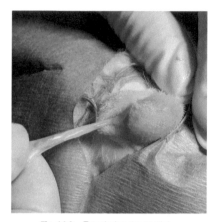

Fig. 14.8 Exteriorize the testicle.

Remove Fat

Fat is removed from along the spermatic cord by sliding a clamp cranially along the cord. Fat can cause the knots tied in the cords to not tighten sufficiently, thereby causing them to come untied and bleed postoperatively (Fig. 14.9).

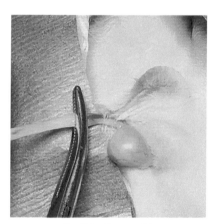

Fig. 14.9 Remove fat.

PERFORM AUTO-LIGATIONS

- Tie the knot
  Each cord is tied on itself with an overhand or figure-eight knot (surgeon's preference) (Fig. 14.10).
- Slide the knot Cranially
  The knot is slid as far cranially as possible. This enables the surgeon to transect the spermatic cord cranial to the pampiniform plexus. Incising the pampiniform plexus can lead to postoperative bleeding (Fig. 14.11).
- Grasp the Spermatic Cord
  The clamp is rotated 180 degrees and used to grasp the spermatic cord distal to the knot (Fig. 14.12).
- Transect the Cord
  The cord is transected at least 1/8 inch distal to the knot and the testicle is removed. The cord is pulled back through the knot. The knot is checked to be sure it is tight (Figs. 14.13 and 14.14).
- Tighten the knot
  Be sure the knot is secure by gently tugging on the cut end of the spermatic cord.

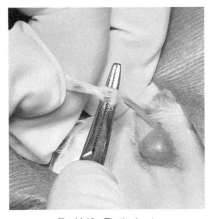

Fig. 14.10   Tie the knot.

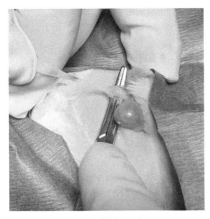

Fig. 14.11   Slide the knot.

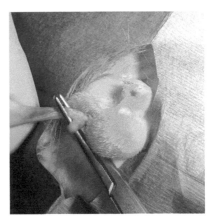

Fig. 14.12   Grasp the cord.

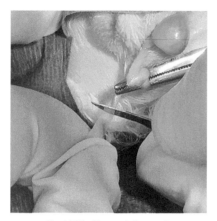

Fig. 14.13 Transect the cord.

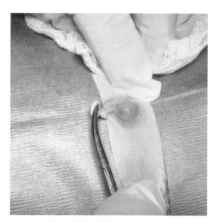

Fig. 14.14 Tighten the knot.

Repeat for the Other Testicle

Elevate the Scrotum

Any fat or remnants of the cord caught in the skin incision will interfere with healing. While holding the skin incision together, the scrotum is gently pulled up to cause any extraneous tissues to be retracted back into the body and away from the incision (Fig. 14.15).

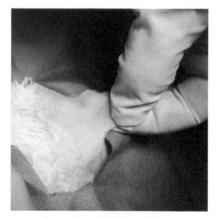

Fig. 14.15 Elevate the scrotum.

Allow to heal by Second Intention

The scrotal incision is not closed.

Consider a Tattoo in Kittens less than 4 Months old

To prevent unnecessary surgery in the future, consider applying a dot of green ink to the caudal end of the scrotal incision. Dab surgical glue over just the ink to prevent staining of the owner's clothes, car, etc. Do not allow the glue to close the scrotal incision.

TROUBLESHOOTING

Fluid in the Scrotum

- Normal in Juveniles
  Ascites is "normal" in kittens due to the hypoproteinemia frequently present in young animals. Abdominal fluid can be transferred from the abdomen to the scrotum via the inguinal canal.
- Recommend Appropriate Diet
  Owners should be advised that if they are not already doing so, they need to feed good-quality kitten food.

CHAPTER 15

Inguinal Cryptorchid Neuter

Victoria Valdez, DVM

There are many protocols for removing a retained testicle from the inguinal area. I use a protocol that uses manipulation of the testicle to the prescrotal midline. The advantage of this technique is that it saves time because there is only one incision to close. It only takes a little longer than a standard prescrotal neuter.

The inguinal testicle is located by manual palpation. It is often easy to mistake a muscle belly or a lymph node for a testicle. If it is not clear, try palpating the same area on the noncryptorchid side of the patient. If a similar mass is palpable on that side, it is probably a muscle or a lymph node. I continue only when I am sure I can palpate the testicle and that I can manually push it close to the prescrotal midline. (If the testicle can not be moved within reach of the midline, see "Troubleshooting" below.) Once these criteria are met, I use the following protocol for an Inguinal Cryptorchid Neuter.

PROTOCOL

Locate the Cryptorchid Testicle by Palpation

In the example pictured (Fig. 15.1), the retained testicle is visible in the right inguinal area. This is not always the case. It often resides deeper in the inguinal canal and can only be located by palpation. Be sure that you can manually move the testicle close to the midline incision.

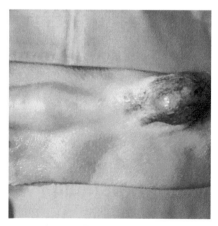

Fig. 15.1 Right retained testicle.

Remove the Nonretained Testicle

The scrotal testicle is removed first via a prescrotal incision in canines. This establishes the location of the canine prescrotal midline incision. (Fig. 15.2) is showing the prescrotal midline incision with the scrotal testicle removed.

In felines, the nonretained testicle is removed via a scrotal incision.

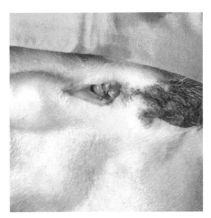

Fig. 15.2   Scrotal testicle removed.

If Needed, Make a Prescrotal Midline Incision

This is necessary in all felines and in bilaterally cryptorchid canines. The skin is pulled toward the surgeon (to avoid the underlying urethra), and it is incised along the midline. The incision must be long enough to extrude the testicle through it. Note: The incision should be a little larger than the cross-sectional diameter of the testicle. It does not have to be as long as the longitudinal length of the testicle.

Manually Relocate the Testicle

The cryptorchid testicle is manually pushed as close to the midline incision as possible (Fig. 15.3).

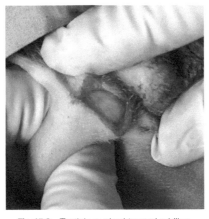

Fig. 15.3   Testicle pushed toward midline.

Expose the Retained Testicle

The testicle is held in place next to the midline, and a *shallow* incision is made from the midline incision to the area over the testicle (Figs. 15.4 and 15.5).

While still applying pressure to hold the testicle in place, blunt dissection is used to free it from its surrounding tissue (Fig. 15.6).

It is sometimes helpful to grasp the testicle with a clamp once it is sufficiently exposed (Fig. 15.7).

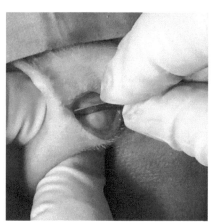

Fig. 15.4   Incise over the testicle.

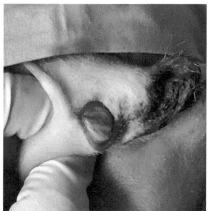

Fig. 15.5   Expose the testicle.

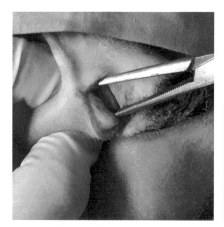

Fig. 15.6   Blunt dissection.

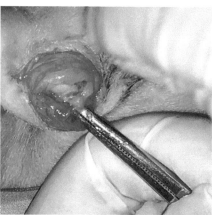

Fig. 15.7   Grasp testicle.

Exteriorize the Retained Testicle

Blunt dissection is continued until the testicle can be exteriorized either by pushing it through the incision manually or by pulling it through the incision with the clamp (Figs. 15.8 and 15.9).

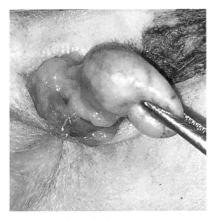

Fig. 15.8 Further exposure.

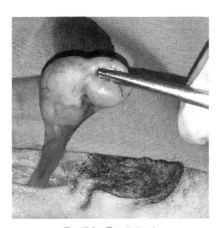

Fig. 15.9 Exteriorized.

Ligate the Spermatic cord using a Miller's Knot

Use a Miller's knot of 2-0 chromic gut.

- Make a Loop in the Suture
  Using an approximate 8 in of suture, a 4-in loop is made in the suture. The loop is placed on the far side of the part requiring ligation (Fig. 15.10).
- Place One Tail Through the Loop
  One tail of the suture is placed through the loop and grasped with needle holders (Fig. 15.11).
- Place the Suture
  The suture is slid to the desired location on the spermatic cord, near the body (Fig. 15.12).
- Tighten the First Ligature
  Pulling the two tails of the suture in opposite directions secures the first of the two ligatures formed by one Miller's knot (Fig. 15.13).
- Adjust Placement for Second Ligature
  The tails of the suture are placed up in an inverted V formation to aid in forming the bump between the two ligatures of the knot, prior to tying the second ligature (Fig. 15.14).
- Tie Second Ligature
  The second ligature is tied leaving space between it and the first ligature, so that a bump is formed between the two (Fig. 15.15).
- Complete the Knot
  The knot is completed with three throws, and the sutures are clipped (Fig. 15.16).

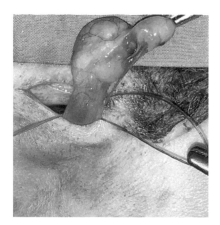

Fig. 15.10 Placing the loop.

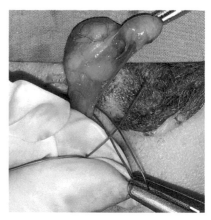

Fig. 15.11 Tail through the loop.

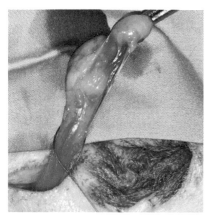

Fig. 15.12 Placement.

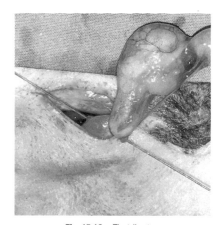

Fig. 15.13 First ligature.

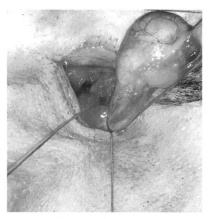

Fig. 15.14 Adjust ties.

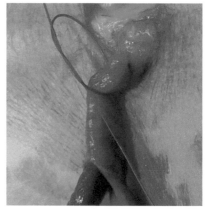

Fig. 15.15 Second ligature.

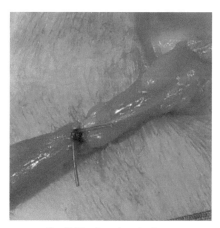

Fig. 15.16   Complete the knot.

Close the Incisions

- Close the Peritesticular Incisions
  The peritesticular incisions are closed with one continuous suture pattern of 2-0 polydioxanone with just one knot. The closure is started with a simple continuous pattern to close the peritesticular incisions, with sutures placed beginning in the far edge of the left peritesticular incision, through the midline to the far edge of the right periesticular incision and repeats until those incisions are closed (Figs. 15.17 and 15.18).
- Close the Skin
  Without placing a knot, the same suture is then used to close the skin in a subcuticular pattern. The first bite starts deep and comes up in the subcuticular tissue, just under the skin. The next bite crosses to the other side of the incision and travels in the opposite direction. It starts and ends in the subcuticular tissue. The last bite crosses back to the near side of the incision and starts in the subcuticular tissue but ends deep (Figs. 15.19–15-21) below. For security, an extra throw is added to the knot (for a total of five throws).

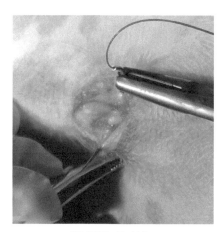

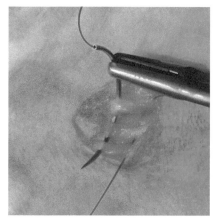

Fig. 15.17   First bite.   **Fig. 15.18**   Additional bites.

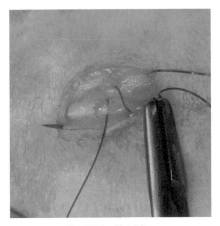

Fig. 15.19 First bite.

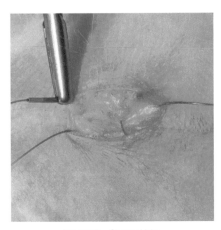

Fig. 15.20 Second bite.

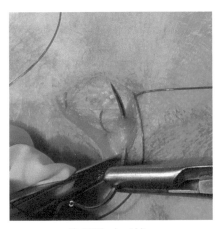

Fig 15.21 Last bite.

Consider Applying a Tattoo

A small dot of green tattoo ink is applied to the cranial portion of the skin incision (the opposite end of the incision from where the knot is). Tattooing the patient helps to prevent an unnecessary abdominal exploratory in the future and the inherent risks associated with it.

Apply Tissue Glue to the Skin

Tissue glue is applied to the skin, being careful to cover the tattoo ink so that it will not stain the owner's car, clothes, and furniture. Also, for extra safety, a drop of glue is placed on the subcuticular suture's knot to make it more secure.

TROUBLESHOOTING

Unable to move Retained Testicle Sufficiently close to Midline

- Verify That It Is a Testicle

  If you are not able to move the testicle to the midline, consider that it may not be a testicle. A lymph node or a muscle belly can feel like a testicle. The contralateral side is palpated to check for a similar-feeling mass. If a like one exists on the nonretained side, they probably are not testicles.

- Do a Cut-Down If Necessary

  If it really is a testicle and cannot be moved sufficiently, the testicle is held in situ and a cut-down is done over it.

- Close the Inguinal Incision(s)

  The peritesticular incision is closed with 2-0 polydioxanone in a continuous pattern. The subcuticular tissue is closed with 2-0 polydioxanone in a subcuticular pattern. If cut-down approaches were made bilaterally, the tattoo is placed in a short, shallow incision in the prescrotal area, since that is the area that will be checked for the presence of testicles. Tissue glue is used to seal the skin.

- Close the Prescrotal Incision, If Indicated

  The prescrotal midline incision is closed as described earlier.

CHAPTER 16

Abdominal Cryptorchid Neuter

Victoria Valdez, DVM

If only one testicle is palpable in an animal, it is probably a unilateral cryptorchid. If both testicles are not palpable in a cat or dog, it has either already been neutered or it is a bilateral cryptorchid. Assuming the patient has NOT been neutered previously, if one or both testicles are retained, they may be abdominal or anywhere along the inguinal canal. If the testicle is in the inguinal canal lateral to the prescrotal area, it is possible to do an inguinal cryptorchid neuter as outlined in the previous chapter. If the testicle is not in the scrotum and not palpable in the inguinal area, it is most likely in the abdomen. Another possibility is that the testicle is so high in the inguinal canal, it is very difficult or impossible to palpate. I have found that, for me, the best approach to find the testicle in either of the two latter scenarios is with an abdominal approach. It may seem like a waste of time to open the abdomen to find a high inguinal testicle, but in my experience, it is usually faster in the long run. From the abdomen, gently follow the ductus deferens. If it disappears into the internal inguinal ring, undrape the external inguinal area and watch that area as you very gently tug on the duct. You may be able to see the testicle move, revealing its location. From there you can incise over the area and bluntly dissect down to the testicle and remove it as described in the inguinal cryptorchid neuter protocol.

I use the bladder as my landmark for finding a retained testicle in the abdomen, The approach to the bladder in a cat is straight forward. An approximately 1.5 in (3.8 cm) incision is made over the bladder area, taking care to avoid the bladder. Once the abdomen is opened and the bladder located, the protocol for a feline is essentially the same as that described here for a canine.

Because of the location of the penis in a canine, locating and exteriorizing the bladder is not quite so easy.

There are various approaches to the abdomen of a canine for the purpose of retrieving an abdominal testicle.

I prefer a peripreputial approach with exteriorizing of the bladder. If the testicle is actually free within the abdomen (i.e., not high in the canal), this approach takes about the same time it takes to do a spay of a canine of the same size.

What follows is the protocol I use for an abdominal cryptorchid neuter. The procedure is the same for a cat except a ventral midline incision is made over the area of the bladder rather than a peripreputial one.

PROTOCOL

Express The Bladder

The bladder is expressed prior to the surgical preparation and scrub. Since the bladder is to be exteriorized, emptying the bladder allows for a smaller abdominal incision.

Position The Patient

The patient is placed in dorsal recumbency. The surgeon stands on the right side of the patient regardless of which side the retained testicle is on.

Retract The Penis

In a canine, a towel clamp is used to retract the penile opening away from the abdominal incision, i.e., toward the left side of the dog (Fig. 16.1).

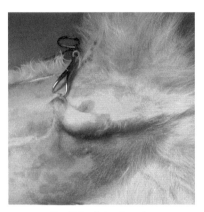

Fig. 16.1 Retract penis.

Make The Ventral Skin Incision

In a canine, a right preprputial incision is made as close to the ventral midline as possible. The right caudal nipple, lateral to the prepuce, is used as a landmark for where to center the incision. The incision should be long enough that the bladder can be exteriorized and the bifurcation of the ductus deferens can be visualized (Fig. 16.2).

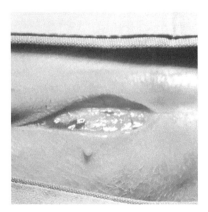

Fig. 16.2 Skin incision.

Make The Abdominal Incision

- Undermine Down to the Abdominal Wall
  The tissue is undermined from the preprputial skin incision to the midline (Fig. 16.3).
- Incise the Capsule
  The capsule of the underlying abdominal muscle is incised (Fig. 16.4).

■ Bluntly dissect into the abdomen

Blunt dissection is used to separate the muscle and enter the abdomen (Fig. 16.5).

In a cat, a ventral midline incision, roughly 1.5 inches long, is made over the bladder area. The surgical blade is held with the sharp edge up to avoid incising the bladder.

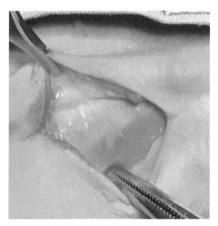

Fig. 16.3   Undermine.

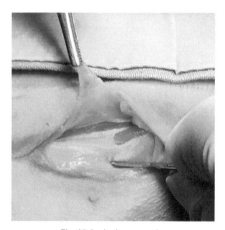

Fig. 16.4   Incise capsule.

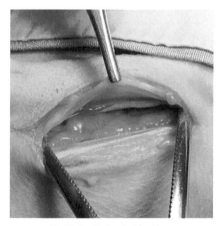

Fig. 16.5   Abdominal incision.

Exteriorize The Bladder

The bladder is located and exteriorized. A stay suture is placed in the apex of the bladder. A clamp is attached to the suture and is used to retract the bladder away from the incision (Fig. 16.6).

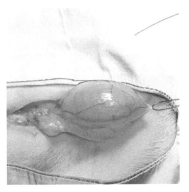

Fig. 16.6   Exteriorize bladder.

Locate The Bifurcation of The Ductus Deferens

The bifurcation of the ductus deferens is located (Fig. 16.7).

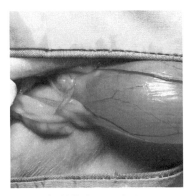

Fig. 16.7   Locate ductus.

Trace The Ductus Deferens To The Retained Testicle

The duct is followed, on the side that is cryptorchid, to the retained testicle (Fig. 16.8).

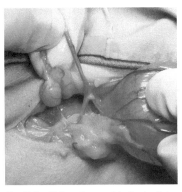

Fig. 16.8   Follow the cord to the testicle.

Exteriorize The Retained Testicle and Remove The Vaginal Tunic

The testicle is exteriorized. In figure 16.9 the structures attached to the testicle read left to right, spermatic cord, ductus deferens, vaginal tunic. The vaginal tunic is manually detached from the testicle. It is usually not necessary to ligate it (Fig. 16.9).

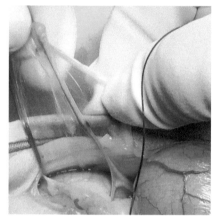

Fig. 16.9   Exteriorize testicle/remove tunic.

Ligate The Spermatic Cord and Ductus Deferens

It is necessary to do an OPEN castration from this point; i.e., the spermatic cord is ligated separately from the ductus deferens. A Miller's knot of 2-0 chromic gut is used for each of the ligatures (Fig. 16.10).

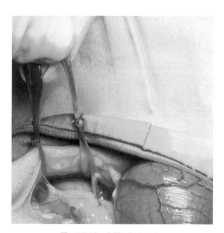

Fig. 16.10   Miller's knots.

Transect The Spermatic Cord and The Ductus Deferens

The spermatic cord and ductus are transected, and the testicle is removed. Repeat for the other testicle if the patient is a bilateral cryptorchid (Fig. 16.11).

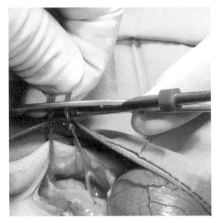

Fig. 16.11   Transect.

Return Cord and Ductus to Abdomen

The bladder and the remnants of the spermatic cord and ductus are replaced into the abdominal cavity (Fig. 16.12).

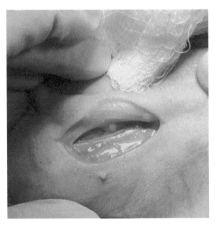

Fig. 16.12   Return the cord to the Abdomen.

Close The Abdominal Incision

Close the abdominal incision in a continuous cruciate pattern with polydioxanone. This pattern begins and ends in the same place, so it requires just one knot. For security, add one or two extra throws to the knot.

Close The Skin

Close the skin with polydioxanone in a continuous subcuticular pattern with just one knot. For security, add an extra throw to the knot and be sure a drop of surgical glue is applied to it. Tissue glue is applied to seal the incision.

Consider Applying a Tattoo

In the canine, a small dot of green tattoo ink is applied to a separate short shallow skin incision in the prescrotal area. Tattooing the patient helps to prevent an unnecessary abdominal exploratory in the future and the inherent risks associated with it.

Apply Tissue Glue

Tissue glue is applied to the skin, being careful to cover the tattoo ink so that it will not stain the owner's car, clothes, and furniture.

Remove The Other Testicle

If the patient is a unilateral cryptorchid and still has one testicle in the scrotum, that testicle is removed via either a prescrotal or scrotal approach, as indicated by the species or age of the patient.

TROUBLESHOOTING

The Cryptorchid Testicle Cannot be Located in the Abdomen

- Do Not Dissect Into the Internal Inguinal Ring From the Abdomen
  There are times when a retained testicle cannot be located in the abdomen. If the ductus deferens disappears into the internal inguinal ring and the testicle is not visible in the inguinal area when it is tugged on, or the ductus breaks at its attachment to the testicle, DO NOT DISSECT into the inguinal ring. This can lead to an inguinal hernia postoperatively. Even more devastating, intractable bleeding can occur, or major nerves can become entrapped in ligatures that are used to stop the bleeding.
- If the Ductus Deferens Breaks
  If the ductus deferens breaks at its attachment to the testicle, and the testicle is out of sight, somewhere in the inguinal canal, it cannot be retrieved from the abdomen. The vessels and ductus are ligated as described above and the area of the *external* inguinal ring is explored for the retained testicle.
- Dissect Down to the External Inguinal Ring
  Blunt dissection is used to separate the subcutaneous tissues from the area of the peripreputial incision to the area overlying the external inguinal ring.
- Locate the Retained Testicle
  The testicle is located, and the duct and vessels are ligated as detailed above.
- Close the Subcutaneous Tissue
  The subcutaneous tissue is closed with polydioxanone in a continuous pattern as needed to close dead space.
- Close the Skin
  The skin is closed with polydioxanone in a continuous subcuticular pattern and tissue glue is applied.

CHAPTER 17

Ancillary Surgeries (Umbilical Hernia, Dewclaw Removal, Feral Cat Ear Tipping)

Victoria Valdez, DVM

With the typical high-volume spay/neuter daily caseload of 30 or more surgeries, there is not a lot of time for ancillary surgeries such as mass removals or enucleations, for example. Patients in need of these surgeries are usually referred to a full-service hospital. However, short procedures such as a small nonreducible umbilical hernia (containing no abdominal organs) or the removal of nonattached dewclaws are often performed in conjunction with the sterilization surgery. Also ear tipping on feral cats is done routinely.

Doing these procedures at the same time as the sterilization surgeries ensures that the patient need not undergo an unnecessary second round of anesthesia.

The protocols I use are the following.

UMBILICAL HERNIA REPAIR PROTOCOL

In an umbilical hernia it is not enough to just close the defect. The hernial ring must be removed. Otherwise the defect will not close, and the hernia will reoccur. When the ring is excised, it always bleeds but will often stop bleeding quickly without the need to ligate the vessel. This makes it a quick procedure.

Incise the Skin

The skin is incised over the protuberance formed by the hernia exposing the hernial sac (Fig. 17.1). (Note: In this patient the incision is so long because the hernia incision is continuous with the spay incision. Such a long incision is not necessary if the patient is not being spayed.)

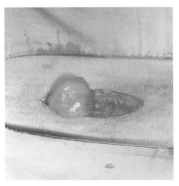

Fig. 17.1 Expose the sac.

Dissect the Hernial Sac

The skin margins are retracted using a 15 blade, and the sac (which is extremely thin) is dissected from the skin edges. This will expose the falciform fat caught in the hernia (Fig. 17.2).

- Identify the Hernia Ring
  Once the sac is completely dissected, slight tension on the falciform fat will reveal the hernial ring (Fig. 17.3).
- Excise the Hernial Ring
  The hernial ring is removed 360 degrees around the protruding fat (Figs. 17.4 and 17.5).

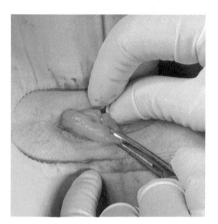

Fig. 17.2   Expose the fat.

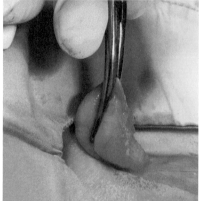

Fig. 17.3   Expose the ring.

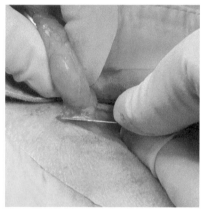

Fig. 17.4   Begin excising the ring.

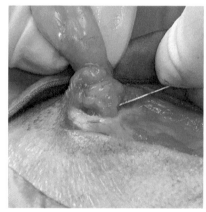

Fig. 17.5   Excise the ring 360 degrees.

Remove or Replace the Falciform Fat

Small amounts of falciform fat, without any adhesions, are inverted back into the abdomen. If this is not possible, the neck of the herniated fat is ligated and the fat distal to the ligature is removed. The ligated fat is returned to the abdomen.

- Check the Hernial Ring for Bleeding
  The site is checked for bleeding. Vessels are ligated as needed.

Close the Hernial Ring

The hernial ring is closed with a 2-0 polydioxanone cruciate suture (Fig. 17.6).

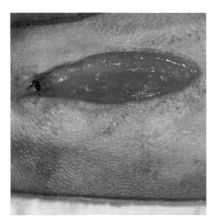

Fig. 17.6 Close the ring.

Close the Skin

The skin is closed with 2-0 polydioxanone with a subcuticular mattress suture and surgical glue.

NONATTACHED DEWCLAW REMOVAL PROTOCOL

Attached dewclaws, especially in a large dog, take time to remove and often require bandaging and, therefore, rechecks. Their removal is best left for another time, if at all. I have developed a protocol I am happy with for removing nonattached dewclaws that is fast, heals well, and does not require skin sutures or bandaging.

Clamp the Base of the Dewclaw

A clamp is placed across the base of the nonattached dewclaw. This is best done before the sterilization surgery and left on during the surgery (Fig. 17.7).

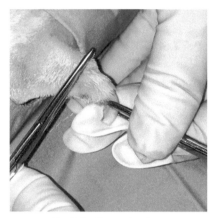

Fig. 17.7   Clamp dewclaw.

Excise the Dewclaw

A blade is drawn directly along the outer edge of the clamp to excise the dewclaw. All extra skin is excised (Fig. 17.8).

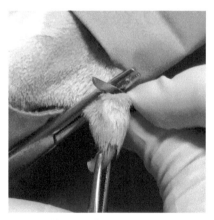

Fig. 17.8   Excise dewclaw.

Apply Epinephrine

With the clamp still in place, epinephrine is applied to the skin edges to constrict the small vessels in the skin. It is allowed to dry for a few seconds. A gauze sponge is used to blot the skin edges dry (Fig. 17.9).

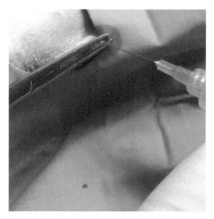

Fig. 17.9 Apply epinephrine.

Apply Surgical Glue to Skin Edges

With the clamp still in place, surgical glue is applied to the skin edges. Excess glue is blotted off the clamp. The glue is allowed to dry a few seconds (Fig. 17.10).

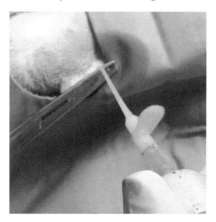

Fig. 17.10 Glue the edges.

Glue the Skin Plantar-Medial to the Clamp

Glue is applied to the skin plantar-medial to the clamp (Fig. 17.11).

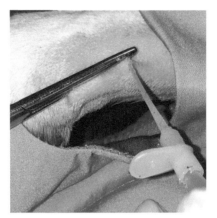

Fig. 17.11   Glue medially.

Fold the Skin over the Glue

The skin (still in the clamp) is folded medially over the glue (Fig. 17.12).

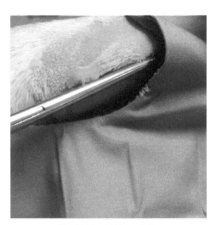

Fig. 17.12   Fold medially.

Remove the Clamp and Hold in Place While the Glue Dries

The clamp is removed while the skin is held in place until the glue dries (Fig 17.13). The thumb is carefully rolled medially to remove it from the glue. Any glove fragments that may have adhered are removed with a clamp.

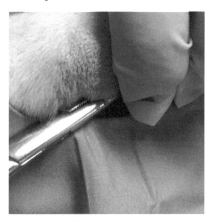

Fig. 17.13 Hold in place.

Clean the Clamp

Using the edge of the surgical blade, any residual glue is removed from the clamp.

Skin Sutures or Bandages are not Needed

Skin sutures and/or bandages should not be necessary but should always be used if indicated.

EAR TIPPING OF FERAL CATS PROTOCOL

Ear tipping is done to establish a visual means of identifying if a cat has already been sterilized. The goal is that a trapped cat does not have to go through the trauma of transportation to the veterinarian if it is already sterilized.

Induce Anesthesia

Cats must be in a surgical plane of anesthesia before their ears are tipped. If they are too light their blood pressure will be too high, and they will bleed post-operatively.

Clamp the Ear

A *straight* clamp is placed across the pinna of the ear about 1/2 inch down from the tip in an adult cat (Fig. 17.14). A proportionate amount of the ear is excised in kittens. A *curved* clamp is not used because a convex cut can be mistaken for a normal ear and a concave cut can be mistaken for a bite wound.

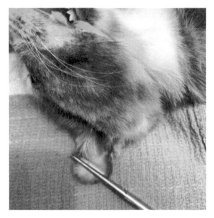

Fig. 17.14   Clamp ear.

Excise the Ear Tip

A blade is drawn directly along the outer edge of the clamp to excise the ear tip. All extra skin is excised (Fig. 17.15).

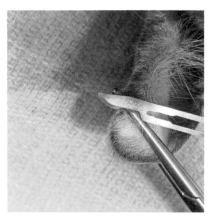

Fig. 17.15   Excise ear tip.

Apply Epinephrine

With the clamp still in place, epinephrine is applied to the skin edges to constrict the small vessels in the skin (Fig. 17.16).

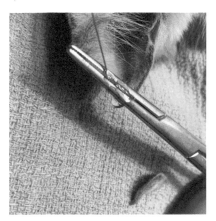

Fig. 17.16 Apply epinephrine.

Apply Styptic Powder

While the epinephrine is still wet, styptic powder is applied to the skin edges with a gauze sponge or cotton-tipped applicator (Fig. 17.17)

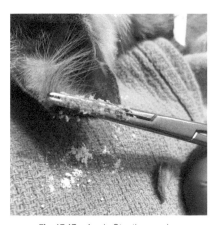

Fig. 17.17 Apply Styptic powder.

Remove the Clamp

Allow the skin to dry for a few seconds, then remove the clamp (Fig. 17.18).

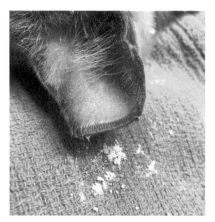

Fig. 17.18 Remove the clamp.

OTHER CONSIDERATIONS REGARDING EAR TIPPING

The Size of the Ear Tip

Sometimes trappers will request, especially for kittens, that the ear tip be "small." This is not recommended because it defeats the purpose of doing it at all. If the kittens are small and can be tamed, a better solution is for the trappers to not have them ear-tipped at all, and to establish a network of volunteers who will tame them and find them homes. If that is not possible and the kittens are to be re-released into the wild, their ear tips need to be readily identifiable.

The Locaiton of the Ear Tip

There is disagreement among animal welfare groups as to which ear should be tipped. From a practical standpoint, if either ear is tipped, that should be a clear indication that the cat has been sterilized. Consult with the groups in your area to see which ear is used for tipping most prevalently, then establish your protocol and be consistent.

Ways To Avoid Ear Tipping The Wrong Cat

Feral cat sterilization surgeries should be done in a block after owned cats are done. This helps to prevent the spread of disease from feral cats to owned cats. This also makes it less likely that an owned cat will be mistaken for a feral cat and inadvertently ear tipped.

On owned cats, a piece of adhesive tape can be applied to the ear that is usually tipped, to alert the surgeon that the ear should not be tipped. Everyone on staff, especially new employees and contract veterinarians should be made aware of the protocols used to avoid ear tipping owned cats.

Complications

CHAPTER 18

Complications

Victoria Valdez, DVM

In high-volume spay/neuter, every effort is made to avoid complications; however, it is true that the more surgeries that are performed, the greater the number of complications that will be seen. It is important to remember that these happen even to the best of surgeons. When, not if, complications arise, then is not the time for self-recriminations. The important thing is to be prepared and know what to do in these situations. I classify complications as minor if they are relatively easy to correct and have no lasting effect, if caught and corrected early. Some commonly seen relatively minor complications include minor damage to the spleen, abdominal bleeding, or scrotal hematomas. Therefore, protocols are included here to repair minor splenic tears, find and stop abdominal bleeders, and perform a scrotal ablation. The protocols I use to treat these complications are described below. Major complications and how to prepare for them are also addressed in this chapter. Chapter 19 covers the most serious complication we encounter, cardiac arrest.

Splenic Repair Protocol

It is easy to nick the spleen with the surgical blade when the abdominal incision is made, to gouge it with the spay hook when attempting to locate the uterine horn, or even to puncture it with your finger when digitally moving it or other organs. With the advent of hemostatic gels or sponges, it is no longer always mandatory to remove the spleen if this happens. Whether or not a splenectomy is necessary depends on whether or not the bleeding can be controlled.

- Exteriorize the Affected Area

    The spleen or the part of the spleen that is bleeding is exteriorized (Fig. 18.1).

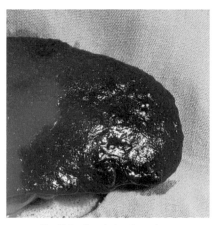

Fig. 18.1   Exteriorize the spleen.

- Apply Epinephrine
  A few drops of epinephrine are instilled in the wound to cause contraction of the spleen (Fig. 18.2).
- Cut the Gel Pad to Size.
  The gel pad is cut to overlap the wound by 1/8 inch at each end (Fig. 18.3).
- Apply Hemostatic Gel Deep
  If the wound is deep hemostatic gel is placed in the crevice of the wound. It is not sutured in place. (If the wound is superficial proceed to the next step).
- Apply Hemostatic Gel to The Surface
  Hemostatic gel is sutured over the wound. 4-0 or finer dissolvable suture is used. The gel must cover the needle tracts placed in the splenic capsule otherwise more bleeding will occur at these sites. A very gentle hand is required to avoid doing further damage to the spleen.
- Tack The Hemostatic Gel in Place
  Mattress sutures are used to hold the hemostatic gel in place. Use only as many sutures as it takes to hold the gel in place.

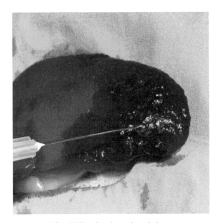

Fig. 18.2 Apply epinephrine.

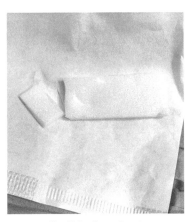

Fig. 18.3 Cut gel pad.

- The First bite with the needle goes through the gel pad (Fig. 18.4)
- Next a shallow bite is taken under the splenic capsule, in this illustration, to the left of the wound Fig 18.5.
- The needle is then brought back up through the gel pad (Fig. 18.6).
- The knots are tied securely, but gently, on top of the gel pad. This helps prevent the suture from cutting through the splenic tissue (Fig 18.7).
- These mattress type sutures are repeated as needed, to secure the gel in place (Fig. 18.8).

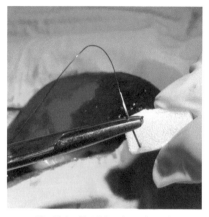

Fig. 18.4   First bite through gel.

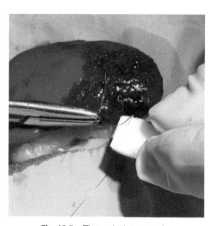

Fig. 18.5   Through the capsule.

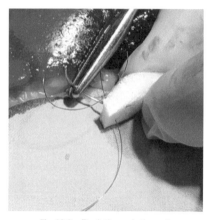

Fig. 18.6   Back through the gel.

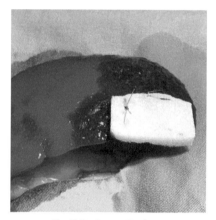

Fig. 18.7   Secure the knot.

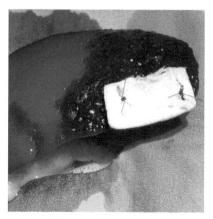

Fig. 18.8   Repeat sutures as needed.

- Cover the Affected Part of the Spleen With Omentum
  The omentum is placed around the affected part of the spleen. It is not sutured in place, as this could cause further bleeding from the spleen (Fig. 18.9).
- Close the Abdomen
  A standard abdominal closure is used.
- Perform Splenectomy If Needed
  If hemostasis cannot be achieved, a splenectomy must be performed. See discussion of major complications below.

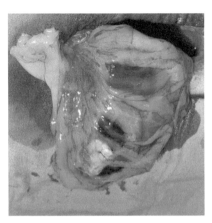

Fig. 18.9 Omentum cover.

Abdominal Bleeding Protocol

This is a life-threatening situation, but completely fixable if found in time. Sometimes, the slipping of spay (or less commonly neuter) ligatures is immediately apparent. Sometimes, it takes astute observation during recovery, or postoperatively, to spot the signs that the patient is in trouble.

Signs to look for are:
- Delayed recovery
- Hypothermia
- Pale mucous membranes
- Weakness
- Bleeding from the incision site may or may not be present
- Free blood in the abdomen found on abdominocentesis (note: absence of or failure to find blood on abdominocentesis does not rule out its presence)
- WHEN IN DOUBT, GO BACK IN.

Prepare for Surgery
- An intravenous (IV) catheter is placed, and the patient is given shock doses of IV fluids.
- Extend the Abdominal Incision
  The abdominal incision is extended so it is long enough that the surgeon can reach into the abdomen and feel the location of the kidneys, as well as retrieve and exteriorize the uterine stump.
- Remove Blood
  Suction or lap sponges are used to remove as much blood as is necessary to determine the source of the hemorrhage. Alternatively, if the hemorrhage is so rapid the source cannot be determined, a methodical inspection of possible sources is begun.

- Rule Out a Splenic Bleed
  If the hemorrhage is rapid, it is often a splenic wound. The spleen is inspected for possible damage. If the spleen is bleeding, it is repaired as detailed earlier. Then the ovarian pedicles and uterine stump are located, and inspected as described below.
- Locate and Inspect the Ovarian Pedicles
  The left pedicle is easier to find than the right, so it is explored first. The colon is retracted toward the midline.
  The location of the left kidney is palpated. The pedicle is in the connective tissue just caudal to the kidney. The pedicle is manually exteriorized, checked for bleeding, and ligated as needed. It is possible for the pedicle to bleed when it is free in the abdomen but not bleed when it is under the tension of being exteriorized. Therefore, even if the ligature is in place, the pedicle is ligated cranial to the original ligature in case the vessels migrated cranially. A retaining suture is placed in the stump and is replaced into the abdomen and checked for bleeding. If no bleeding is seen the retaining suture is removed. The same steps are repeated with the right side, using the duodenum as the retractor. Care is taken to manipulate the pancreas as little as possible to avoid subsequent pancreatitis.
- Locate and Inspect the Uterine Stump
  The bladder is located and exteriorized. The uterine stump is located between the bladder and colon, and exteriorized. The uterine stump is inspected to determine if the ligature is in place. It is possible for the stump to bleed when it is free in the abdomen but not bleed when it is under the tension of being exteriorized. Therefore, even if the ligature is in place, the arteries on either side of the uterus are individually ligated, followed by a ligature around the entire uterus, in the event that the vessels migrated caudally. Place a retaining suture in the stump and replace it in the abdomen and check for bleeding. If no bleeding is seen the retaining suture is removed.
- Remove Residual Blood
  Suction, if available, is used, followed by lap sponges to remove residual blood. The abdomen is checked for any active bleeding. If present, the source is found and dealt with.
- Close the Abdomen
  A standard abdominal closure is used.

Scrotal Ablation Protocol

Scrotal hematomas, post neuter, are quite common. If there is no drainage, these can often be managed medically with cold then hot compresses, analgesics, and drugs to keep the patient quiet. Antibiotics are given if needed. If the area is draining and/or infected, it is often best to do a scrotal ablation. Since the scrotum is in effect redundant skin with respect to the perineal area, there is usually not a problem closing the defect formed by removing the scrotum. A problem could arise if skin surrounding the scrotum has become necrotic due to pressure from swelling. The area should be evaluated prior to surgery. If it appears that an ablation would cause too much tension for a straightforward closure, and the spay/neuter surgeon is not experienced in tension-relieving surgical techniques, the patient should be referred to a surgeon proficient in plastic surgery.

- Position the Patient
  The patient is placed in dorsal recumbency. To avoid tension on the surgery site, the back legs are not tied.
- Make the Incision
  An elliptical incision is made around the base of the scrotum. If the scrotal skin is viable, the incision can be made higher on the scrotum to give the surgeon more skin with which to close.
- Remove the Hematoma and Any Dead Tissue
  Blunt dissection is used to remove the tissues underlying the scrotum. Vessels are carefully ligated or cauterized to achieve hemostasis.

- Close the Incision

  Closure is in three layers, to obliterate dead space. Strong tension-relieving sutures (0 polydioxanone) are used as needed. The subcuticular layer is closed with 2-0 polydioxanone in a subcuticular pattern. Surgical glue is used in the skin or it is closed with the surgeon's preference of skin sutures or staples.

Preparation for Major Complications

Major complications include things like a hemorrhagic spleen, a broken ureter, an incised bowel, or the presence of a diaphragmatic hernia. You may not encounter these complications for years. However, THESE COMPLICATIONS CAN AND DO HAPPEN TO THE BEST OF SURGEONS. The key is to be prepared. These are life-threatening complications that require immediate surgical intervention. Your patient's life depends on your ability to handle these eventualities. If you do not feel qualified to perform a splenectomy, remove a kidney, close an incised bowel loop, or repair a diaphragmatic hernia, you must at the very least know how to stabilize the patient sufficiently to safely transfer that patient to a surgeon who can. However, referral is not always practical or even possible. The best course is for you to thoroughly familiarize yourself with the protocols for the previously mentioned surgeries.

- Invest in Good Veterinary Surgical Texts

  There are numerous veterinary texts that better describe the protocols for these surgeries than can be done here.

- Post Relevant Protocols

  I recommend that after you have familiarized yourself with the protocols for the surgeries mentioned earlier, you post laminated copies of the protocols, along with their illustrations, on the walls of your surgery. They will then be there for review when, not if, the day comes that you need them.

- Create a Binder Containing Pertinent Protocols

  If you are an independent contractor and travel from practice to practice, you may want to carry a binder containing these protocols with you at all times. You never know when they will be needed.

- Be Prepared

  Remember, these complications are RARE. It is not as if you perform these surgeries frequently enough to be fully versed in their execution at a moment's notice. A quick review is always helpful. TAKE A DEEP BREATH AND DO WHAT NEEDS TO BE DONE. There is great satisfaction in handling a crisis like this well, so be prepared.

CHAPTER 19

Cardiac Arrest

Victoria Valdez, DVM

Cardiopulmonary arrest (CPA) is the ultimate complication we encounter in high-volume spay/neuter. It requires all our skill, training, and teamwork in a high-pressure situation. There is no time to learn as we go when every second is critical. Therefore, as with any major complication, we must be prepared. This requires a plan, proper equipment, and continual training. What is your plan?

Who does what, and in what order? What equipment do you need, and where and how will it be stored? How will it be utilized? Does your staff know what to do in the event of cardiac arrest? What about new hires? Are you current on the latest drugs and techniques used in cardiopulmonary resuscitation (CPR)?

There are many protocols used in the event of cardiac arrest. I recommend you use what you are comfortable with. Just be sure your staff are well trained and you have all the drugs and equipment you need. Everyone is more comfortable if they know what to do and are prepared. The example protocol presented here is based on each person having specific duties to perform, but these are guidelines, and each team member can and should step in and help another if one is busy and the other has free time. The following is the protocol I use; it is simply listed here as an example.

CPR PROTOCOL

When an animal goes into cardiac arrest, it is an all hands on deck situation. Everyone on staff should be trained to do all of the positions listed below, since various staff members may be absent when a CPA event occurs. Note this is a protocol based on a team comprised of one doctor, one licensed or registered technician, one prep person and one recovery person. Your staff may vary. You should develop a protocol that fits your individual resources and needs. For the following example protocol, there should be a person assigned to each of the following positions: ventilation, chest compressions, drug administration, and patient monitoring. The duties of each position are listed below. All duties should be performed as simultaneously as possible.

Positions

- Ventilation Person

  If CPA occurs while the patient is under anesthesia, the anesthetic agent should be turned off, and oxygen delivery maintained. Any drugs that can be, should be reversed.

  Clear the airway, intubate the patient, if not already in place, connect to oxygen, then bag the patient. (Note: I prefer to initially give the patient oxygen by mouth-to-tube or mouth-to-nose, if it is not already intubated. This better allows me to access any resistance in the endotracheal tube or the lungs. The American Veterinary Medical Association [AVMA] recommends one mouth-to-snout ventilation for every 15 chest compressions. If I feel resistance to ventilation, I pull the tube to check for blood or mucus that may be interfering with the passage of oxygen, then place a clean tube.) It is critical that oxygen perfusion to the brain be restarted as soon as possible, i.e., even before the heart is restarted, if necessary. We have all had those patients for whom we have successfully restarted the heart but hypoxia has caused irreparable brain damage. I continue oxygen delivery in this manner until the tongue is pink and then switch to manual bagging. The AVMA CPR guidelines recommend that intubated dogs and cats be ventilated manually at a rate of 10 breaths per minute, i.e., one breath every 6 seconds. The bag should be squeezed to a pressure of 10–15 cm H_2O.

■ Chest Compressions Relief Person

Once started, chest compressions are not stopped until the heart is beating strongly on its own. The AVMA recommends compressions be performed at a rate of 100–120 beats per minute (BPM). To approximate these rates, the song "Stayin' Alive" has a beat of 103 BPM. Singing or humming to this song while doing compressions may help establish the correct rhythm needed.

The patient is placed in lateral recumbency (except for barrel-chested dogs, such as bull-dogs), with its back facing the person doing the compressions. In medium, large, and giant-breed dogs, it may be necessary for the person doing the compressions to stand on a stool in order to place the compression provider's shoulders directly over the patient and get the degree of compression necessary to achieve adequate perfusion. After each compression, the chest is allowed to recoil to its normal size and shape. For all but cats and toy breed dogs, the hands of the person doing the compressions are placed one on top of the other with the elbows locked. Where this person places his or her hands on the patient depends on the size and chest conformation of the patient. The following recommendations are based on guidelines published by RECOVER (Reassessment Campaign on Veterinary Resuscitation), a joint project produced by the Veterinary Emergency and Critical Care Society (VECCS) and the American College of Veterinary Emergency and Critical Care (ACVECC).

■ Round-Chested Dogs.

In round-chested dogs, i.e., those whose chests are as wide as they are long, the thoracic pump method is used. The hands are centered on the widest part of the chest cavity and the chest is compressed one-third to one-half its depth. The goal is to apply intrathoracic pressure to the thoracic vasculature sufficient to create forward blood flow.

■ Deep-Chested Dogs.

In narrow-chested dogs, i.e., those whose chests are narrower than they are wide, the cardio pump method is employed. In this method, the hands are placed over the heart. Each compression physically pushes blood out of the heart, and it is allowed to refill as the chest recoils.

■ Barrel-Chested Dogs.

In dogs with barrel chests, i.e., those whose chest is wider than it is deep, the dog should be placed in *dorsal recumbency* with the hands placed over the sternum (i.e., the heart) to utilize the cardiac pump method.

■ Toy Breeds and Cats.

In toy breeds and cats, one hand is placed around the chest with the thumb over the heart on the upmost side and the fingers on the opposite side of the chest. Compression of the heart between the thumb and fingers (by one-third the chest size) utilizes the cardiac pump method.

Whichever method is used, studies have found that the provider becomes fatigued after 2 minutes. For this reason, this position should be rotated among available staff every 2 minutes. Therefore, one person (a relief person) is needed to rotate from one position after another, relieving the person in that position so that they may take their turn doing chest compressions.

■ Drug Administration Person

A table of Emergency Drug Dosages is kept with the crash cart/kit and posted at each anesthetic machine. A sample table is included below. For ease in calculation dosages are in mls per 10lbs (5kgs) and tables are provided in 5lb (~2.5kg) increments. Drugs should be given intravenously if at all possible. Drugs are listed in order of use i.e., the order in which they are pulled up. For example, pre-med reversal drugs are the first needed followed by atropine or epinephrine. All drug administration is done under the doctor's direction.

Administer vasopressors such as epinephrine every 3–5 minutes during CPR.

Pull drugs up for endotracheal administration prior to beginning catheter placement. Endotracheal cardiac drugs may be delivered via a red rubber catheter placed in the endotracheal tube. The drug dosages are doubled for endotracheal administration. The drug is flushed into the endotracheal tube followed by a breath of air either by mouth-to-tube or by bagging the patient to push the drug into the lungs.

Syringes should be labeled with the first letter of the drug to prevent confusing them. It may take a minute or two for the doctor to ascertain if atropine or epinephrine is the drug needed. Pull up both, label them, then be sure the doctor knows which is which.

An intravenous (IV) catheter should be placed as soon as possible. Preferably, everyone on staff should be proficient in placing a catheter. Because of decreased blood pressure in the CPA patient, it is usually necessary to place a smaller-gauge catheter than would normally be appropriate. Once an IV catheter is placed, IV drug administration can begin (Table 19.1).

Note: Only drugs used for reversal, atropine, and epinephrine are shown on this Table; you may want to add other drugs such as those used to treat cardiac arrhythmia or shock. Fluid administration rates may also be a helpful addition to this chart.

TABLE 19.1 ■ Emergency Drugs in mL/5 lb Body Weight Increments

Weight in Pounds	Weight in Kilograms	Naloxone 0.4 mg/mL 0.04 mg/kg	Flumazenil 0.1 mg/mL 0.01 mg/kg	Atipamezole 5 mg/mL 0.05 mg/kg	Atropine 0.54 mg/mL 0.05 mg/kg	Epinephrine[a] 1:1000 0.01 mg/kg Low Dose	0.1 mg/kg High Dose
5	~2.5	0.25 mL	0.25 mL	0.02 mL	0.25 mL	0.02 mL	0.25 mL
10	~5	0.5 mL	0.5 mL	0.05 mL	0.5 mL	0.05 mL	0.5 mL
15	~7.5	0.75 mL	0.75 mL	0.75 mL	0.7 mL	0.07 mL	0.7 mL
20	~10	1.0 mL	1.0 mL	0.1 mL	1.0 mL	0.1 mL	1.0 mL
25	~12.5	1.25 mL	1.25 mL	0.12 mL	1.2 mL	0.12 mL	1.2 mL
30	~15	1.5 mL	1.5 mL	0.15 mL	1.5 mL	0.15 mL	1.5 mL
35	~17.5	1.75 mL	1.75 mL	0.17 mL	1.7 mL	0.17 mL	1.7 mL
40	~20	2.0 mL	2.0 mL	0.2 mL	2.0 mL	0.2 mL	2.0 mL
45	~22.5	2.25 mL	2.25 mL	0.22 mL	2.2 mL	0.22 mL	2.2 mL
50	~25	2.5 mL	2.5 mL	0.25 mL	2.5 mL	0.25 mL	2.5 mL

TABLE 19.1 ■ Emergency Drugs in mL/5 lb Body Weight Increments—cont'd

Weight in Pounds	Weight in Kilograms	Naloxone 0.4 mg/mL 0.04 mg/kg	Flumazenil 0.1 mg/mL 0.01 mg/kg	Atipamezole 5 mg/mL 0.05 mg/kg	Atropine 0.54 mg/mL 0.05 mg/kg	Epinephrine[a] 1:1000	
						0.01 mg/kg Low Dose	0.1 mg/kg High Dose
55	~27.5	2.75 mL	2.75 mL	0.27 mL	2.7 mL	0.27 mL	2.7 mL
60	~30	3.0 mL	3.0 mL	0.3 mL	3.0 mL	0.3 mL	3.0 mL
65	~32.5	3.25 mL	3.25 mL	0.32 mL	3.2 mL	0.32 mL	3.2 mL
70	~35	3.5 mL	3.5 mL	0.35 mL	3.5 mL	0.35 mL	3.5 mL
75	~37.5	3.75 mL	3.75 mL	0.37 mL	3.75 mL	0.37 mL	3.75 mL
80	~40	4.0 mL	4.0 mL	0.4 mL	4.0 mL	0.4 mL	4.0 mL
85	~42.5	4.25 mL	4.25 mL	0.42 mL	4.2 mL	0.42 mL	4.2 mL
90	~45	4.5 mL	4.5 mL	0.45 mL	4.5 mL	0.45 mL	4.5 mL
95	~47.5	4.75 mL	4.75 mL	0.47 mL	4.7 mL	0.47 mL	4.7 mL
100	~50	5.0 mL	5.0 mL	0.5 mL	5.0 mL	0.5 mL	5.0 mL

Drug dosages are doubled for endotracheal administration.
[a]Low-dose epinephrine is recommended for routine use every 3–5 minutes. High-dose epinephrine may be considered after prolonged cardiopulmonary resuscitation.

■ Patient Monitor

A good stethoscope is procured immediately for the doctor to auscult the patient's heart for the presence of asystole. The patient is hooked up to a pulse oximeter for the purpose of monitoring the heat rate and SpO_2 of the patient. If a pulse oximeter is not available, the stethoscope is used frequently to determine the heart rate of the patient.

The patient's temperature is taken to check for hypothermia. Hypothermia can be fatal and happens rapidly, especially in very small animals. It is important to keep them warm, but staff should be well trained in the safe use and precautions associated with the use of heating devices in the treatment of recumbent patients to prevent associated burns and hyperthermia. If fluid bottles are heated in the microwave to be used as hot water bottles, they must be hot enough to transfer heat to the patient but not so hot that they burn. The person preparing the bottles should hold them against his or her underarm for a count of 10 seconds to make sure they are not too hot. The hot water bottle should always be wrapped in a towel or fleece before being set against the patient. Electrical heating pads are notorious for short-circuiting or creating hot spots. The patient's body should be frequently checked in areas where it is in contact with the heating pad for any hot spots. When using a hair dryer to warm a patient, the highest setting should never be used. If waving it directly over the patient, the person operating the hair dryer should hold his or her splayed fingers over the animal in the path of the hot air to be sure it is not too hot. The patient's temperature is checked frequently for evidence that it is returning to normal and that it is not overheating.

Note: Since CPA events frequently involve a patient in recovery, there is often another patient on the table undergoing surgery as this takes place. There could also be a third patient under anesthesia on the preparation table. If all anesthetic machines are in use, the animal in preparation needs to be recovered while resuscitation efforts are performed on the CPA patient. The surgery site of the surgery patient needs to be covered with a sterile drape or towel. Someone needs to at least periodically monitor the stability of the other patients on the surgery table and in recovery (or preparation). The person monitoring the CPA patient should be able to monitor the other anesthetized patients once CPR is underway.

ASSIGNMENTS

The staff is allowed to choose what position each wants to perform in a CPR event as long as they can demonstrate that they are proficient in all of them. For example, they may position themselves as follows:

Chest Compressions Relief Person: Doctor
Drug Administration: Registered or Licensed Technician
Patient Monitoring: The Recovery Person
Ventilation: The Prep Person

Variation to the above: As the doctor, I prefer to start with the ventilation position so I can personally assess resistance to air flow in the lungs or endotracheal tube. Therefore, I start the ventilation person in the chest compression position while I start ventilation. After 2 minutes, I switch with the person doing chest compressions. Once that switch is made, everyone is in their "permanent" positions as listed earlier. I then switch with each person in turn so they may have a turn doing chest compressions. When they have done CPR for 2 minutes, they return to their "permanent" positions. The cycle is repeated until the patient is resuscitated or time of death is called.

CRASH CART

Replenish the crash cart after every use. Once the CPR is concluded, one person needs to be responsible for being sure it is restocked. The most efficient person to do this is the person who was in charge of drug administration, since he or she is most likely to know what was used from the crash cart/kit.

Crash Cart Maintenance

- Laminated List
  A laminated list of required contents should be part of the cart or kit.
- Crash Cart Contents
  Table 19.2 shows what the minimum content of the cart should be.

TABLE 19.2 ■ **Crash Cart/Kit Contents**

Equipment for Placing Catheters	Equipment for Administering Drugs	Drugs (Based on Doctor's Preference)
All available sized intravenous catheters	All available size hypodermic needles	Appropriate reversal drugs
Male adapter plugs	Preneedle capped syringes	Atropine
Butterfly catheters: all sizes	Size 1.0 cc	Epinephrine or vasopressin
Size 15 surgical blades	Size 3.0 cc	Cardiac arrhythmia drugs
Gauze	Syringes in a variety of other sizes	Dopram
Adhesive tape	Prefilled saline flush syringes, 3.0 cc	Dex-SP
Antibiotic ointment (eye lube)		Others as desired

- Personalize Cart
  Personalize this chart to meet your preferences.
- Label Crash Cart Contents
  Each compartment in the crash cart/kit should be clearly labeled as to what belongs in it.
- Label Crash Cart Location.
  If the crash kit is kept in a cupboard, the cupboard should be labeled with the words "CRASH CART" in large letters and everyone should be made aware of its location.

TRAINING

Staff CPR refresher training should be held a minimum of twice a year or whenever a new person is hired, if possible. Alternatively, a training video showing your CPR protocol could be made and shown to new hires.

Everyone on staff needs to be trained in the following:

- The location of crash cart and its contents
- How to estimate the patient's weight
- How to calculate or refer to the drug dosage chart to determine drug doses based on the patient's weight
- How to place a rear leg catheter in dogs and cats
- Positioning and technique for chest compressions
- How to maintain the proper rhythm for chest compressions
- How to use the anesthesia machine to ventilate the patient
- How to monitor the CPA patient
- How to operate the pulse oximeter
- How to auscult the heart
- The proper use of heating devices
- How to stock the crash cart/kit.

The doctor should keep abreast of the latest drugs, dosages, and techniques used in CPR and any changes in guidelines published by appropriate veterinary organizations.

Page numbers followed by "*f*" indicate figures, "*t*" indicate tables.

NOTES

NOTES